AF887467

Cardiovascular Pathophysiology for Pre-Clinical Students

Instructor Resources

How to Adopt This Book

This is an open textbook. That means that this book is freely available and you are welcome to use, adapt, and share this book with attribution according to the Creative Commons NonCommercial ShareAlike 4.0 (CC BY-NC-SA 4.0) license https://creativecommons.org/licenses/by-nc-sa/4.0. (Many, but not all images, illustrations, etc in this book are licensed under CC BY 4.0.)

Instructors reviewing, adopting, or adapting this textbook are encouraged to register at https://bit.ly/interest-preclinical. This assists the Open Education Initiative at Virginia Tech in assessing the impact of the book and allows us to more easily alert instructors of additional resources, features and opportunities.

Finding Additional Resources for Your Course

The main landing page for the book is https://doi.org/10.21061/cardiovascularpathophysiology.

This page includes:

- Links to multiple electronic versions of the textbook (PDF, ePub, HTML)
- Links to the instructor resource-sharing portal
- Link to errata document (report errors at https://bit.ly/feedback-preclinical)
- Links to other books within this series

Sharing Resources You've Created

Have you created any supplementary materials for use with Cardiovascular Pathophysiology for Pre-Clinical Students such as presentation slides, activities, test items, or a question bank? If so, please consider sharing your materials related to this open textbook. Please tell us about resources you wish to share by using this form: https://bit.ly/interest-preclinical or by directly sharing resources under an open license to the public-facing instructor sharing portal https://www.oercommons.org/groups/pre-clinical-resources/10133.

Customizing This Book

The Creative Commons Attribution NonCommercial-ShareAlike 4.0 license https://creativecommons.org/licenses/by-nc-sa/4.0/legalcode on this book allows customization and redistribution which is NonCommercial, that is "not primarily intended for or directed towards commercial advantage or monetary compensation."

Best practices for attribution are provided at https://wiki.creativecommons.org/wiki/ Best_practices_for_attribution.

This book is hosted in PDF and ePub in VTechWorks http://hdl.handle.net/10919/105409 in HTML in Pressbooks https://pressbooks.lib.vt.edu/cardiovascularpathophysiology and via the LibreTexts platform https://med.libretexts.org/@go/page/34347. Pressbooks and LibreTexts platforms both offer customization/remixing.

Cardiovascular Pathophysiology for Pre-Clinical Students

ANDREW BINKS

PDF AND EPUB FREE ONLINE AT: HTTPS://DOI.ORG/10.21061/CARDIOVASCULARPATHOPHYSIOLOGY

VTC | Virginia Tech Carilion School of Medicine

VIRGINIA TECH PUBLISHING

VIRGINIA TECH CARILION SCHOOL OF MEDICINE IN ASSOCIATION WITH VIRGINIA TECH PUBLISHING
BLACKSBURG, VA

Suggested citation: Binks, Andrew (2022). Cardiovascular Pathophysiology for Pre-Clinical Students. Roanoke: Virginia Tech Carilion School of Medicine. https://doi.org/10.21061/cardiovascularpathophysiology. Licensed with CC BY-NC-SA 4.0 https://creativecommons.org/licenses/by-nc-sa/4.0.

Publisher: This work is published by the Virginia Tech Carilion School of Medicine in association with Virginia Tech Publishing, a division of the University Libraries at Virginia Tech.

Virginia Tech Carilion School of Medicine 2 Riverside Circle Roanoke, VA 24016 USA

Virginia Tech Publishing University Libraries at Virginia Tech 560 Drillfield Drive Blacksburg, VA 24061 USA https://publishing.vt.edu publishing@vt.edu

This work is also distributed by LibreTexts, Davis, CA USA info@libretexts.org. Note: The LibreTexts version of this work at https://med.libretexts.org/@go/page/34347 may differ from this version.

Peer review: This book has undergone single-blind peer review by two external reviewers.

Accessibility statement: Virginia Tech Publishing is committed to making its publications accessible in accordance with the Americans with Disabilities Act of 1990. The Pressbooks (HTML) and ePub versions of this text are tagged structurally and include alternative text, which allows for machine readability.

Publication cataloging information:
Binks, Andrew, author
Cardiovascular Pathophysiology for Pre-Clinical Students / Andrew Binks
Pages cm
ISBN 978-1-957213-02-6 (PDF)
ISBN 978-1-957213-03-3 (ePub)
ISBN 978-1-957213-01-9 (Pressbooks) https://pressbooks.lib.vt.edu/cardiovascularpathophysiology
ISBN 978-1-957213-04-0 (Print)
URI (Universal Resource Identifier) http://hdl.handle.net/10919/105409
DOI https://doi.org/10.21061/cardiovascularpathophysiology

1. Cardiovascular system – Pathophysiology
2. Cardiovascular system – Diseases I.
   Title RC669.9 .B56 2022

Disclaimer: The information in this textbook is intended for educational purposes only and is not meant to take the place of medical care, diagnoses, or services. Please see your healthcare provider about any health concerns.

Cover art: Kindred Grey, CC BY 4.0
Illustration and cover design: Kindred Grey

Contents

Introduction

Cardiovascular disease is one of the prevalent clinical issues that graduating health care professionals will address. The purpose of this book is to provide an understanding of the basic concepts of common diseases of the cardiovascular system in preparation for professional exams and the clinic.

Cardiovascular Pathophysiology for Pre-Clinical Students, is an undergraduate medical-level resource for foundational knowledge of common cardiovascular diseases, disorders and pathologies. This text is designed for a course pre-clinical undergraduate medical curriculum and it is aligned to USMLE(r) (United States Medical Licensing Examination) content guidelines. The text is meant to provide the essential information from these content areas in a concise format that would allow learner preparation to engage in an active classroom. Clinical correlates and additional application of content is intended to be provided in the classroom experience. The text assumes that the students will have an understanding of basic cardiovascular physiology that will be helpful to understand the content presented here. This resource should be assistive to the learner later in medical school and for exam preparation given the material is presented in a succinct manner, with a focus on high-yield concepts.

Cardiovascular Pathophysiology for Pre-Clinical Students is intended to address both necessary content and align with the preclerkship curricular needs. The utility of a flexible text can positively impact the learning environment and increase student engagement and performance. This text is made to be adaptable by using pieces and parts to suit students and inspire the addition of elements to this living resource.

Features of this Book

- Detailed learning objectives are provided at the beginning of each subsection
- High resolution, color contrasting figures illustrate concepts, relationships, and processes throughout
- Summary tables display detailed information
- Accessibility features including structured heads and alternative-text provide access for readers accessing the work via a screen-reader

This resource was designed to fill a gap in undergraduate medical education (UME) and support preclerkship education in the content areas of basic science for medical education. Unlike traditional textbooks, the organization of this resource is driven by curricular structure, rather than subject area. As the format and design of UME differs across many programs, this resource is purposefully brief and flexible, allowing for rapid adaptation across programs. The resource is organized into small chapters that can be used to support student preparation in any arrangement. The sections are not intended to be all-inclusive, but rather primers for applied content delivery. In our curriculum, these topic areas are interwoven into problem-based and case based learning modalities. The cases and clinical correlates change regularly and having the flexibility of these short resources that can be applied to many scenarios across the pre-clinical years of our curriculum is beneficial.

Over the past twenty years, medical education has undergone a rapid curricular restructuring. This is in part due to recommendations of the Flexner report[1], coupled with the changes observed in millennial[2] and iGen learners. To accommodate the integration of additional core competencies, the majority of medical programs have moved away from discipline-based delivery and currently use some form of integrated curricular format.[3] This allows material to be presented in a more clinically realistic and pertinent format without the constraints of artificial discipline silos. This movement has had positive impacts on programmatic outcomes and student performance, but it has presented some challenges for curricular design, student engagement and educational resources.

Although contemporary medical curricula have moved to a cohesive, integrated format, the required textbooks for undergraduate medical education remain traditional and discipline-based. Use of small, independent chapters allows content to be delivered in a variety of curricular settings and support content integration and alignment.

A high volume of content, some of it lacking alignment with class sessions coupled with restrictions on student contact time imposed by accrediting bodies, means that faculty across the country are having to rethink preparation materials to facilitate efficient, focused learning experiences. This resource It is intended to provide learners with a high-level view of relevant topical areas that will be further elaborated on within the classroom setting. Unlike other traditional textbooks, it is not intended to include all content a learner would need about the relevant subject area but to function as a stepping stone towards mastery of the content.

As programs embrace the philosophy of student-directed learning embedded in adult learning theory, more simplified readily available resources will be essential to support this fast-paced learning of health professional educational programs. While there are many factors that can contribute to a student's lack of preparation, lengthy textbook resources for a single integrated classroom session have a significant negative impact. So while an integrated curricular model enhances many aspects of learning, it makes using traditional textbooks cumbersome and disjointed for students. This resource hopes to address this concern.

Finally, there is a wealth of "medical" content freely accessible online, and students can find themselves spending a significant amount of time trying to identify alternative resources that may—or may not—be appropriate. Faculty taking ownership to identify and adapt realistic materials for each session reduces the concern that students are finding misinformation through internet sources, and this project allows faculty to create a resource that harnesses the best attributes of many different formats into a product that best supports the learning environment. Otherwise, external online resources are also likely to contain extraneous content that is not aligned with the classroom learning objectives (akin to subject-based textbook chapters), so it can also reduce the perceived worth of preparation. If the integrated resource is generated correctly, concisely and accurately by the faculty, the students will gain trust, rely on the vetted resources and prepare for the active classroom.

References

1. Cooke M, Irby DM, Ph D, et al. American Medical Education 100 Years after the Flexner Report. 2006:1339-1344.
2. Roberts DH, Newman LR, Schwartzstein RM. Twelve tips for facilitating Millennials' learning. Medical Teacher. 2012;34:274-278.
3. VanTassel-Baska J, Wood S. The integrated curriculum model (ICM). Learning and Individual Differences. 2010;20(4):345-357.

About the Author and Acknowledgments

About the Author

Dr. Andrew Binks is a cardiopulmonary physiologist who gained his BSc (Hons) in Physiological Sciences at the University of Newcastle upon Tyne, then a MSc in Human and Applied Physiology from King's College, London. He returned to Newcastle to do his PhD and study the underlying physiological mechanisms of dyspnea, the cardinal symptom of cardiopulmonary disease. He continued investigating dyspnea at Harvard School of Public Health as a postdoctoral fellow and then as a research scientist. After seven years at Harvard, Andrew took his first faculty position at the University of New England where he taught cardiovascular and pulmonary physiology to health profession and medical students. He continued to teach medical students their heart and lung physiology after moving to the University of South Carolina's Medical School in Greenville where he also directed the school's heart and lung pathophysiology courses. Andrew currently teaches heart and lung physiology and pathophysiology at Virginia Tech Carilion School of Medicine, directs the heart and lung pathophysiology course and has also served as the departmental director of faculty development.

In his two decades of teaching medical physiology, Andrew has regularly drawn upon his dyspnea research experience to generate an active, clinically focused approach to medical education. This book is part of that approach and supports students preparing for class with the basic information with the intention to apply and contextualize that information in a guided case-based classroom experience.

Andrew has published numerous peer-reviewed research papers and book chapters about dyspnea and about contemporary medical education. He has also given keynote presentations, faculty workshops and international webinars to promote effective medical education for the modern adult learner.

Acknowledgments

Funding and In-Kind Support
Publication of this work is made possible in part through the support of VIVA (Virtual Library of Virginia), LibreTexts, the Open Education Initiative of the University Libraries at Virginia Tech, and Virginia Tech Publishing.

Peer Reviewers
Lauren Kennedy-Metz, Instructor in Surgery, Harvard Medical School
Anonymous research professor

Editorial Team
Managing Editor: Anita Walz
Graphic Design and Editorial Assistance: Kindred Grey
Alternative Text: Andrew Binks and Sophia DeSimone

Special Thanks
Delmar Larson, Founder, LibreTexts
Christa Miller, Accessible Technologies, Virginia Tech

1. Arrhythmias

Learning Objectives

- Distinguish between different forms of common arrhythmias.
- Describe the underlying pathophysiology of an arrhythmia.

This chapter will address the arrhythmias listed in the USMLE (United States Medical Licensing Exam) Step 1 content guide on a section-by-section basis. Learning the arrhythmias here will be substantially easier with a robust understanding of electrocardiogram (ECG) fundamentals and lead orientation, so going back to basics is likely to be very worthwhile.

Atrial Fibrillation

Atrial fibrillation is the most common cardiac arrhythmia and is caused by rapidly firing potentials in the atrial myocardium. These aberrant depolarizations are often the result of myocardial remodeling and frequently originate within the muscular sleeves that extend into the pulmonary veins from the atria. Causes include hypertension, valvular and ischemic heart disease, and genetics (e.g., mutation of 10q22–q24 on chromosome 10). The rapid depolarizations result in a very fast atrial rate from 400 to 600 bpm. Because the atrial rate is so fast, the ECG shows "coarse fibrillatory waves" (figure 1.1); the action potentials produced are low amplitude, and P-waves will not be seen.

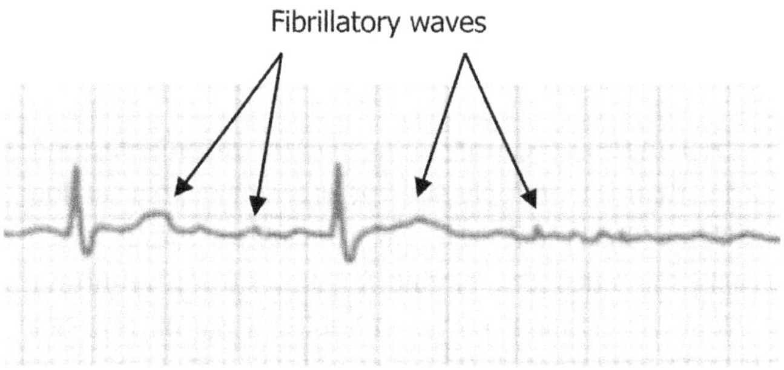

Figure 1.1: An ECG of atrial fibrillation showing lack of P-waves and low-amplitude fibrillation waves between QRS complexes.

The rapid atrial depolarizations are transmitted to the atrioventricular (AV) node, but far from all are conducted through to the ventricle because of the node's long refractory period. This means the ventricular rate does not rise to 400–600 bpm (which would be catastrophic), but some of the atrial fibrillation activity can be "lucky" and reach the AV node when it is not in a refractory period. When this occurs, the ventricular rate rises to 100–200 bpm, and QRS complexes can be "irregularly irregular" with a varying R-R interval (left panel, figure 1.2).

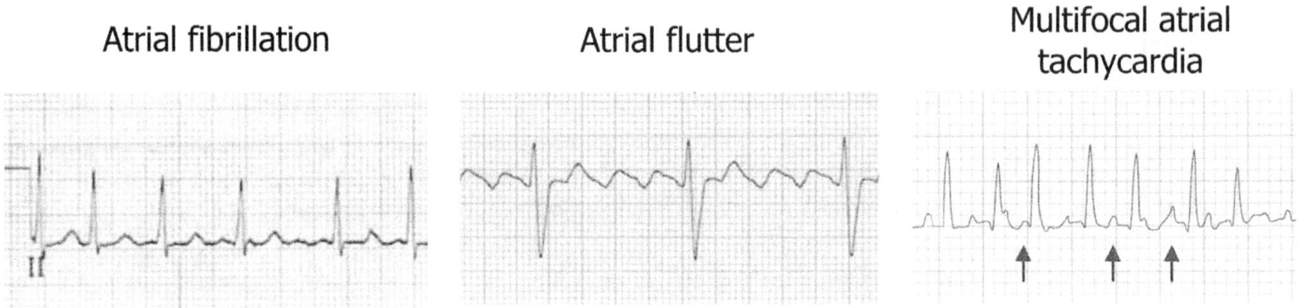

Figure 1.2: Comparison of atrial arrhythmias, including atrial fibrillation (left), atrial flutter (middle), and multifocal atrial tachycardia (MAT) (right).

Atrial fibrillation summary
No visible P-waves
Irregularly irregular QRS complexes
High ventricular rate
Atrial fibrillatory waves possible

Table 1.1: Atrial fibrillation summary.

Atrial Flutter

Atrial flutter is caused by a macroreentrant current, rather than the multiple sites of aberrant depolarization seen in fibrillation. The cavotricuspid isthmus (CTI) usually provides the circuit for the slower reentrant current to become established (typical atrial flutter), but other sites of reentry and slow conducting circuits are possible (atypical atrial flutter) and are usually associated with structural heart disease or sites of previous surgical or ablations procedures. The slower reentry current produces an atrial rate of 250–350 bpm (compared to the 400–600 of atrial flutter), and P-waves are present but have a characteristic "sawtooth" pattern (figure 1.3 and middle panel figure 1.2).

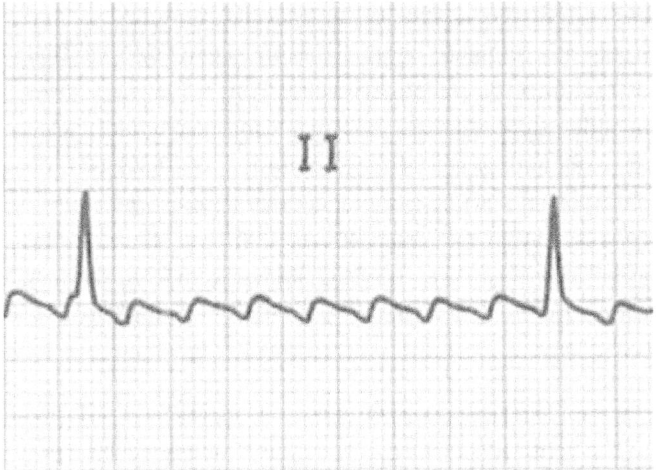

Figure 1.3: Atrial flutter — "sawtooth" P-waves with lower frequency than the fibrillation waves of atrial fibrillation.

As with atrial fibrillation, the AV node's refractory period prevents most of the P-waves from progressing to the ventricle, but commonly the AV conduction will be 2-to-1, so with an atrial rate of 300 bpm the ventricular rate will be 150 bpm. Parasympathetic stimulation or changes in AV node refractoriness can modify how many P-waves pass into the ventricle, but the the resultant rhythm is "regularly irregular." When the heart rate is elevated, then distinguishing flutter from fibrillation becomes challenging and slowing ventricular rate pharmaceutically (adenosine) helps the flutter waves reemerge for a definitive diagnosis to be made.

Atrial flutter summary
Sawtooth atrial pattern
Regularly irregular QRS complexes
High ventricular rate

Table 1.2: Atrial flutter summary.

Multifocal Atrial Tachycardia

Multifocal atrial tachycardia (MAT) is caused by the presence of multiple ectopic foci. The multiple foci result in P-waves with multiple morphologies and irregular intervals (see figure 1.4). The pathophysiology of MAT is not clear, although several theories exists (e.g., triggered activity, reentry, or abnormal automaticity). The multiple foci within the atrium generate consecutive action potentials that are all conducted to the ventricles. Thus, each QRS complex will be preceded by a P-wave; however, each P-wave will have a different morphology because they originate from different areas. By definition, MAT must have at least three distinctly different P-wave morphologies (figure 1.4) and a ventricular rate of greater than 100 bpm.

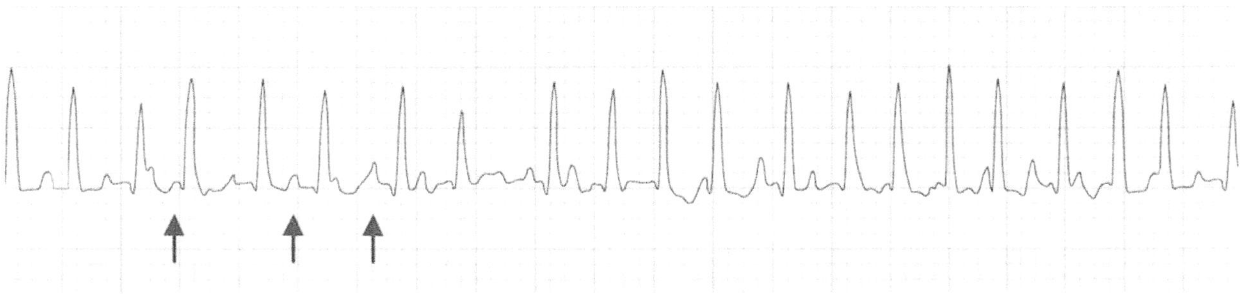

Figure 1.4: Three distinct P-wave morphologies in a case of MAT.

MAT frequently occurs in the setting of severe lung disease and, more specifically, during an exacerbation of lung disease. This rhythm is benign, and once the underlying lung disease is treated, it should resolve.

MAT summary
P-waves followed by QRS complexes
P-waves have different morphology (at least three)
High ventricular rate (100 bpm)

Table 1.3: MAT summary.

Premature Atrial Contraction

A premature atrial contraction (PAC) is generated by a depolarization instigated outside of the SA node. This produces an extra P-wave, and consequently a shortening from previous P-P intervals is seen. The aberrant P-wave also has a different morphology from a sinus P-wave because of its different anatomical origin.

The premature complex may also upset the timing of the SA node, placing it back into a refractory period when it should be depolarizing for its next scheduled beat. This means that a PAC may cause a "compensatory pause" as the SA node restarts its pacemaker depolarization. Consequently the ECG can show "atrial bigeminy" where complexes appear to be in pairs with a normal complex followed by a complex driven by the atrial ectopic activity, then a pause while the SA node begins its depolarization again (see figure 1.5).

If a PAC occurs when the AV node has not yet recovered from its refractory period, the PAC will fail to conduct to the ventricles; meaning the PAC will not be followed by a QRS complex or the ectopic P-R interval will be prolonged. The ECG will show a premature, ectopic P-wave and then no QRS complex afterward. When this occurs along with bigeminy, the ECG can appear as if there is sinus bradycardia.

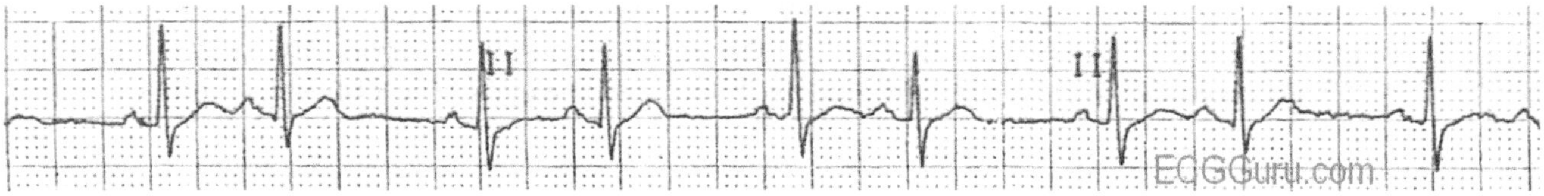

Figure 1.5: Atrial bigeminy in PAC with ECG complexes appearing in pairs.

PAC summary
Extra P-wave with abnormal morphology
Compensatory pause leading to atrial bigeminy

Table 1.4: PAC summary.

Sinus Bradycardia

Sinus bradycardia denotes a sinus rhythm below 60 bpm. Otherwise the ECG waveform is normal on an ECG with an upright P-wave in lead II preceding every QRS complex. There are many intrinsic causes associated with the heart itself, as well as extrinsic causes, some of which are listed table 1.5. Sinus bradycardia is usually asymptomatic as rates of 40–50 bpm can maintain hemodynamic stability. Rates below this can produce symptoms of fatigue, dizziness, and dyspnea on exertion.

Intrinsic causes	**Extrinsic causes**
Chest trauma	Hypothyroidism
Ischemic heart disease	Carotid sinus sensitivity
Sick sinus syndrome	Calcium channel blockers
Myocarditis	Antiarrhythmic class I to IV
Familial disorder	Intracranial hypertension
Radiation therapy	Hypoglycemia
Lyme disease	Sleep apnea

Table 1.5: Intrinsic and extrinsic causes associated with the heart.

Sinus bradycardia summary
60 bpm
Normal P-wave before every QRS complex

Table 1.6: Sinus bradycardia summary.

Premature Ventricular Contractions

Similar to a PAC, a premature ventricular contraction (PVC) occurs when a focus in the ventricle generates an action potential before the pacemaker cells in the SA node depolarize. This early depolarization is out of rhythm with the normal R-R interval, and because it starts outside of the normal conduction pathways, it has a very different shape from a normal, scheduled QRS complex (figure 1.6). The PVC is wider as it has to travel from myocyte to myocyte, so it is much slower than a normal SA node–driven depolarization that travels through the faster conduction network fibers. There is also a compensatory pause following the PVC as the unscheduled depolarization puts the ventricular myocardium into refractory state, forcing it to "skip a beat" (figure 1.6).

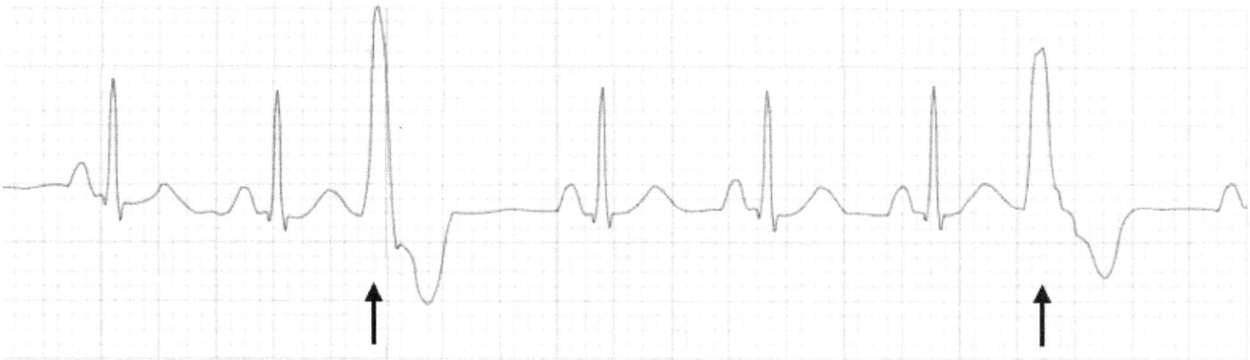

Figure 1.6: PVCs have a wider complex and are followed by a compensatory pause.

PVC summary
Put of step with normal R-R interval
Wider complex
Followed by compensatory pause

Table 1.7: PVC summary.

Ventricular Tachycardia

Ventricular tachycardia (VT) is caused by reentry currents being established in the ventricular myocardium or groups of ventricular myocytes that have aberrant electrical behavior. As such, VT is usually caused by underlying cardiac disease.

Like a PVC, the aberrant depolarizations do not follow the normal conduction pathways so are wide (>120 msecs), but unlike a PVC, VT involves a ventricular rate >100 bpm. With disorganized contractility and reduced filling time, VT can lead to hemodynamic instability and severe hypotension—hence it is life threatening.

The QRS morphology in VT is highly variable between patients and depends on where the arrhythmia originates. Consequently there are several ways to classify VT based on duration, symptoms, QRS morphology, rate, and origin.

Sustained VT is any VT that lasts for more than 30 seconds or is symptomatic. **Nonsustained VT** lasts for less than 30 seconds and is asymptomatic.

VT can be **monomorphic** or **polymorphic** (figure 1.7). The QRS complexes in monomorphic VT have the same shape and are symmetrical because they start in the same place in the myocardium. Polymorphic VT has a variable QRS shape because the depolarizations are instigated at multiple points. An electrophysiologist can describe the location(s) within the ventricles from where the VT originates using the shape(s) of the QRS complexes.

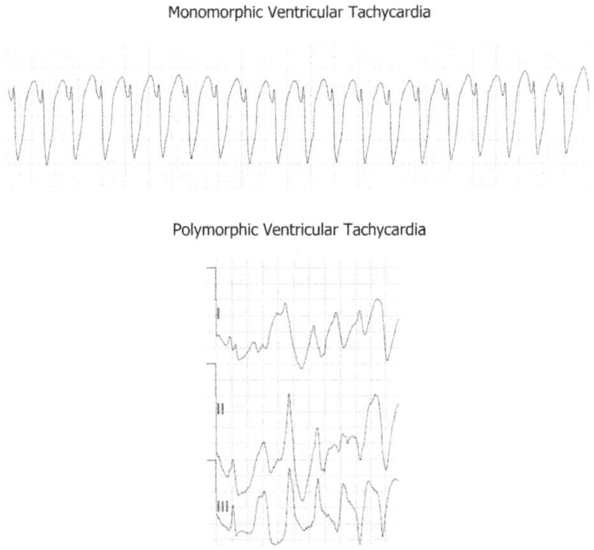

Figure 1.7: Monomorphic and polymorphic VT.

Torsades de pointes (twist of peaks) is a form of VT with multiple QRS morphologies. The twist references the undulating amplitude of the QRS complexes that twist around the isoelectric line, giving the ECG the appearance of a twisted ribbon (figure 1.8).

Torsades de pointes is associated with a prolonged QT interval (>600 msecs) that helps distinguish it from other forms of polymorphous VT. The longer QT interval can be caused by ionic abnormalities that reduce the repolarizing current of Phase 3 of the cardiac action potential. This makes the myocardium susceptible to early after-depolarizations—the trigger for torsades de pointes. These after-depolarizations do not happen uniformly across the myocardium and are more common in endocardial tissue where the repolarization currents are slower. So torsades de pointes arises from the after-depolarizations causing reentry currents in neighboring tissue.

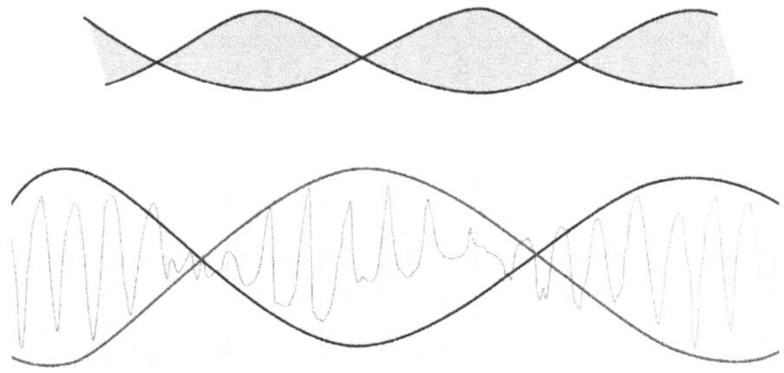

Figure 1.8: Torsades de pointes.

Both common garden variety VTs and torsades de pointes can progress to ventricular fibrillation.

VT summary
Ventricular rate >100 bpm
QRS complex not associated with P-wave
Wide QRS complex morphology

Table 1.8: VT summary.

Ventricular Fibrillation

Ventricular fibrillation (VF) occurs when the ventricular rate exceeds 400 bpm. The disorganized and uncoordinated contraction of the myocardium causes cardiac output to fall to catastrophic levels. Rates of survival for out-of-hospital VF are low.

There are a number of instigating events, but coronary artery disease and resultant myocardial ischemia or tissue scarring are the most common. The onset of VF may be preceded by other changes in the myocardial rhythmicity, such as PVCs, ST changes, VT, or QT prolongation. The tissue damage allows formation of reentry patterns that cause the chaotic ventricular depolarization. These reentry patterns break up into multiple smaller wavelets that cause high-frequency activation of the myocytes. The result is an ECG that is chaotic (figure 1.9) and consequently a heart that has little output.

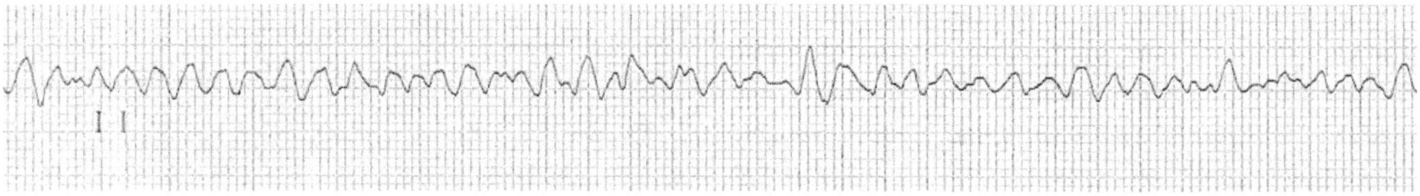

Figure 1.9: Example of VF with no recognizable P-waves or QRS complexes.

VF summary
Chaotic, irregular, and varying intervals
No P-waves, QRS complexes, or T-waves
High rate

Table 1.9: VF summary.

First-Degree Atrioventricular Block

A first-degree atrioventricular node block results from slow action potential conduction through the AV node conduction. The slowing can be due to changes in vagal tone or structural changes associated with damage or disease affecting the conductive tissue of the atria, AV node (most common), bundle of His or bundle branches, and Purkinje system. It takes longer for the action potential to reach the ventricles, so P and R appear further apart. The P-R interval is normally between 0.12 and 0.20 seconds, but in first-degree block it exceeds 0.20 seconds (>5 small boxes; figure 1.10).

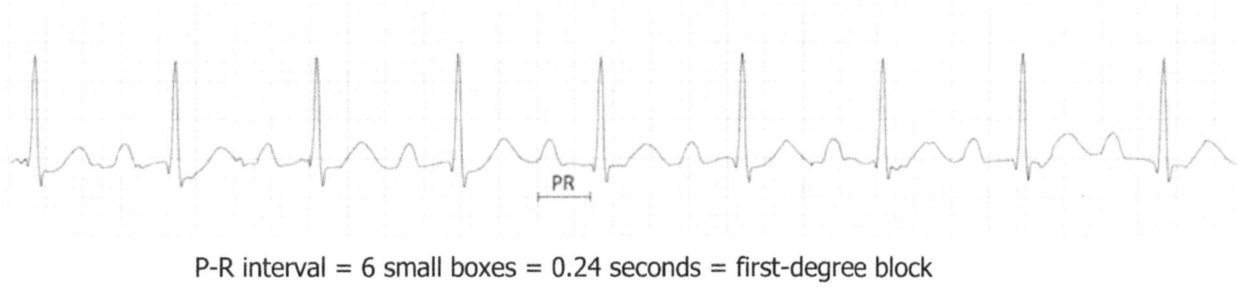

Figure 1.10: Example of first-degree block with P-R interval >0.2 seconds.

In first-degree block each P-wave is accompanied by a QRS complex (i.e., "they all get through") (figure 1.10), which is not the case in second-degree and third-degree blocks (see below). Generally a first-degree block is asymptomatic and does not require any treatment, but long-term monitoring for worsening conduction is advisable.

First-degree block summary
Prolonged P-R interval (>0.2 sec)

Table 1.10: First-degree block summary.

Second-Degree Atrioventricular Block

A second-degree atrioventricular block also has changes in P-R interval, but it starts to show failure of the P-wave to propagate a QRS complex every time (i.e., intermittently the depolarization fails to reach the ventricles). The pattern of missed ventricular depolarizations, or blocked P-waves, is often very regular and described as a ratio of P-waves to QRS complex. The way in which the P-R interval changes in relation to the blocked P-waves produces subclassifications of second-degree blocks, Mobitz I and II.

Mobitz I (or Wenckebach)—The P-R interval progressively lengthens until a P-wave is missed and then goes back to its original length (figure 1.11). So P-R is longest before the dropped QRS complex and shortest immediately after it. This progressive difficulty in traversing the AV node is reflective of the node becoming increasingly refractory.

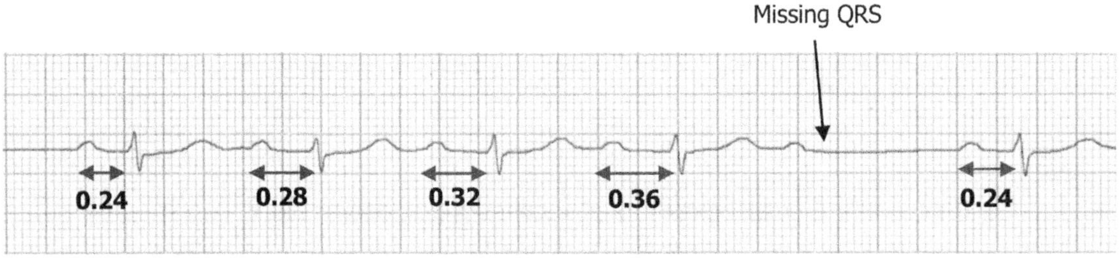

Figure 1.11: Mobitz I (second-degree block) with P-R intervals shown in seconds.

Mobitz II has blocked P-waves as well, but the P-R interval remains unchanged, and the P:QRS ratio appears in a fixed pattern (figure 1.12). This is a rarer and more serious condition and usually involves problems with the conduction system below the AV node, most commonly in the bundle branches. What can frequently been seen is a widening of the QRS complex that are generated.

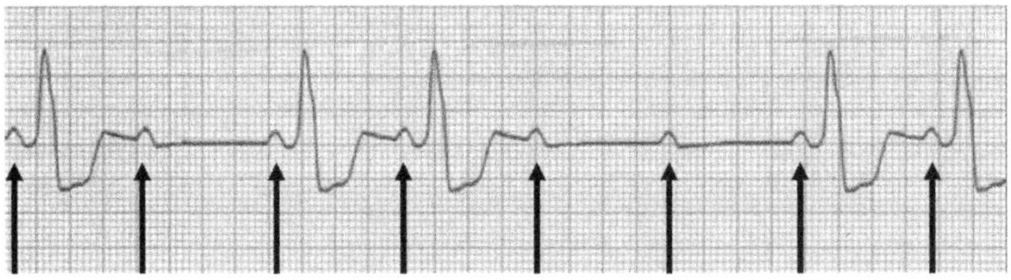

Figure 1.12: Mobitz II (second-degree block) with arrows showing P-waves. The P-R interval is stable, and the ratio is 3:1.

Second-degree block summary
Prolonged P-R interval (>0.2 sec)
Intermittently blocked P-waves
Variable (Mobitz I) or stable (Mobitz II)

Table 1.11: Second-degree block summary.

Third-Degree Atrioventricular Block

A third-degree atrioventricular block is where no action potentials pass through the AV node, hence it is often called "complete heart block". This is usually because of damage (e.g., ischemia) or disease (e.g., Lyme disease, sarcoidosis) affecting the AV node. In a third-degree atrioventricular block, no P-waves have associated QRS complexes. Without any descending control by the SA node pacemakers, the ventricular pacemaker cells are finally free to rule the ventricles (insert maniacal laughter). Consequently P-waves and QRS complexes are completely unrelated to each other, and this is termed "AV dissociation." The ECG (figure 1.13) reflects this with P-waves occurring at an SA node rate (~75 bpm with parasympathetic tone) and the ventricles depolarizing at between thirty and fifty times per minute, depending on which ventricular tissue acts as pacemaker.

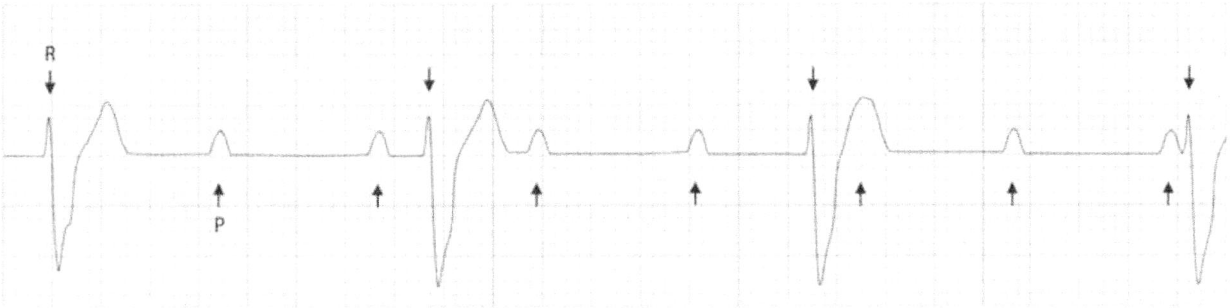

Figure 1.13: Third-degree block with P-waves (black arrows) having an SA node rate of 100 bpm and the ventricles depolarizing (blue arrows) at 33 bpm.

Third-degree block summary
P-waves and QRS complexes dissociated

Table 1.12: Third-degree block summary.

Note:
Prior to reading the next sections, revisit the lead orientations of a 12-lead ECG, and it might be useful to have the normal ECG for comparison.

Left Bundle Branch Block

A left bundle branch block (LBBB) is generated when the conductivity of the His-Purkinje system in the left ventricle is compromised, either through damage or disease. The ECG changes, and criteria for LBBB relate to these changes in conductivity and the left-side location.

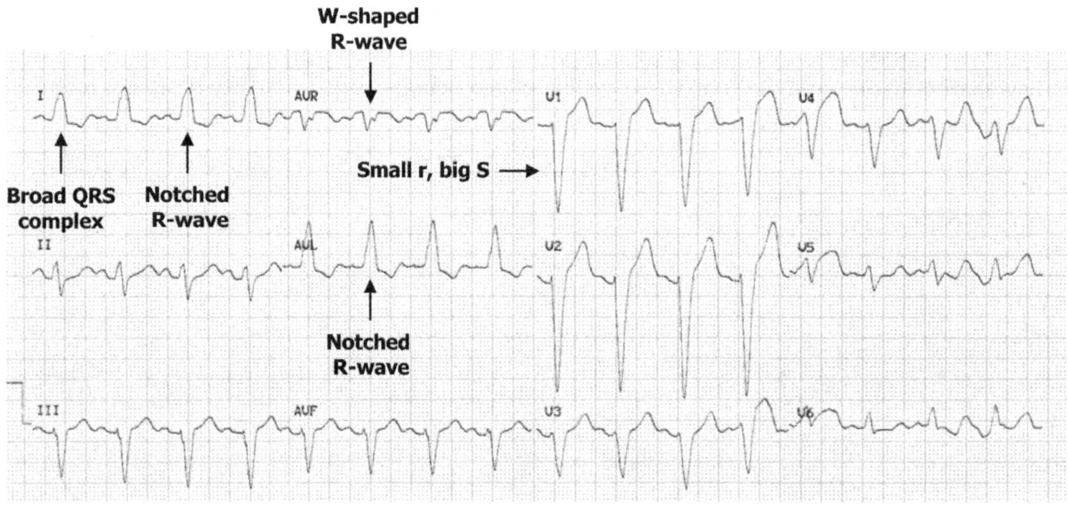

Figure 1.14: Example of LBBB with defining features labeled.

Because the normal route through conductive tissue is impaired or blocked, the depolarization has to travel through myocytes, which takes more time. Consequently, the QRS complex is wider (figure 1.14) (i.e., has a duration >120 msecs, with 80–100 msecs being normal). The slower conduction through the left ventricle means the right ventricle depolarizes first and the left last. This means the depolarization has a prominent right-then-left direction and will be moving away from lead V1, causing that lead to have a deep downward S-wave (figure 1.14).

The lateral leads (I, V5, and V6) normally show a downward deflecting Q-wave as normal septal deflection initially occurs left-to-right (i.e., away from the lateral leads). In LBBB the change in direction to right-to-left, plus the longer duration, eliminates the Q-wave from the lateral leads, and Q-waves will be small in aVL.

The R-wave in the lateral leads may also change morphology when there is a distinct separation of right and then left ventricular depolarization. This manifests as an M-shaped R-wave (figure 1.15) or a notched R-wave in the lateral leads (figure 1.14).

Conversely a W-shaped R-wave may occur in leads facing the opposite direction (e.g., aVR) (figure 1.14).

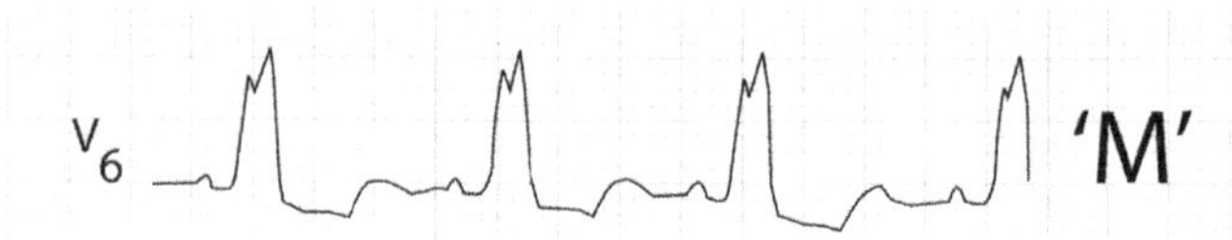

Figure 1.15: Changes in R-wave morphology as differences in left and right depolarization produce an M-shaped wave.

LBBB summary (also see figure 1.14)
QRS complex >120 msecs
Dominant S-wave in V1
Absence of Q-waves in lateral leads

Table 1.13: LBBB summary.

Right Bundle Branch Block

The causes and manifestations of a right bundle branch block (RBBB) bear some similarities to those described for LBBB, but of course this time its depolarization of the right ventricle is delayed. Causes of RBBB include ischemic heart disease again as well as other myocardial diseases, but pulmonary issues such as pulmonary embolism and cor pulmonale can be added to the list.

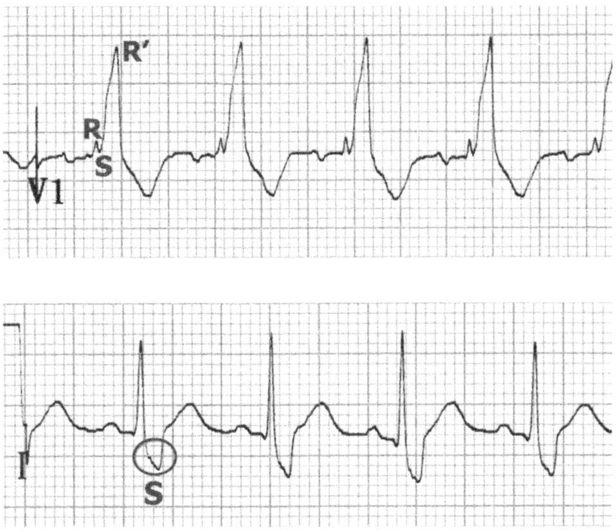

Figure 1.16: Typical RSR' pattern (upper) and slurred S-wave pattern (lower) of RBBB.

Again the QRS complex becomes broad (>120 msecs) because of the slower conduction through ventricular myocytes. However, the delayed activation of the right ventricle causes a secondary R-wave (RSR') to occur in the right precordial leads (V1–V3) and a slurred S-wave in the lateral leads (I, aVL, and frequently V5 and V6) (figure 1.16).

RBBB summary
QRS complex >120 msecs
RSR' pattern in V1–V3
Slurred S-wave in lateral leads

Table 1.14: RBBB summary.

Wolff-Parkinson-White Syndrome

Normally the only electrical connection between the atria and the ventricles is the AV node. Otherwise the fibrous skeleton of the heart electrically insulates the atria from the ventricles. In Wolff-Parkinson-White (WPW) syndrome, that insulation is incomplete, and an "accessory pathway" connects the electrical system of the atria directly to the ventricles. If you think of the AV node as a bridge over the fibrous wall with regulated access, the accessory pathway is like a pathological tunnel under it with no regulation.

The accessory pathway provides a second route (figure 1.17) for normal sinus rhythm to pass from atrium to ventricle much more quickly (there is no AV node delay), thus the P-R interval is shortened. Because of this "preexcitation" through the accessory pathway, the ECG shows a slurring of the onset of the QRS complex, referred to as a delta wave because of its triangular shape (figure 1.18).

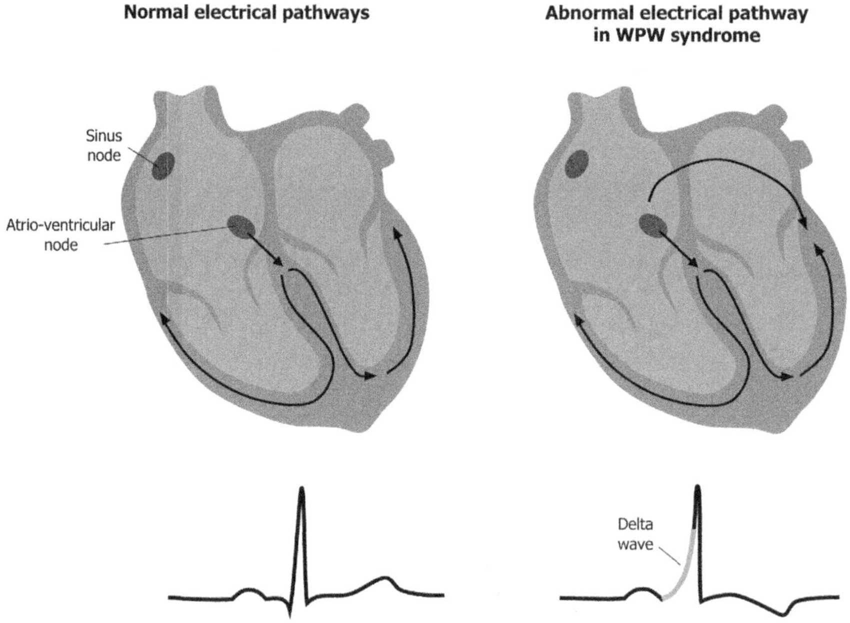

Figure 1.17: Schematics of normal WPW syndrome conductivity pathways.

WPW syndrome is often asymptomatic, and patients do not require immediate treatment. However, if atrial fibrillation occurs in a WPW patient, the accessory pathway can allow the atrial fibrillation waves through to the ventricle (with no AV nodal refractory period to prevent them). Consequently a high ventricular rate is seen, and the risk of ventricular fibrillation being established means immediate clinical attention is required.

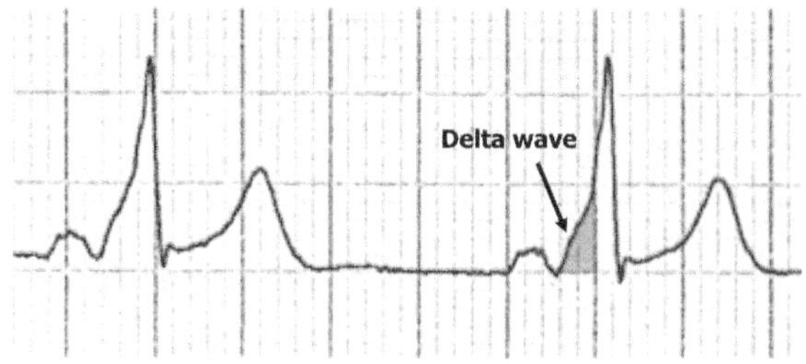

Figure 1.18: Delta wave of WPW syndrome.

WPW syndrome summary
Short P-R interval (120 msecs)
Delta wave slurring the onset of QRS complexes
Broad QRS complexes (>100 msecs)

Figure 1.18: Delta wave of WPW syndrome.

Hyper- and Hypocalcemia

Moderate rises in extracellular levels of Ca^{++} (3.0–3.4 mmol/L, normal = 2.1–2.6 mmol/L) block the movement of sodium through voltage-gated sodium channels. This results in a reduced depolarization of myocytes, and consequently repolarization time is less. Raised extracellular Ca^{++} also changes the closing kinetics of the L-type Ca^{++} channels such that the plateau phase of the cardiac action potential is shortened and repolarization occurs earlier. These two effects manifest as the most common ECG finding of short QT intervals, mainly through shortening of the ST segment (figure 1.19).

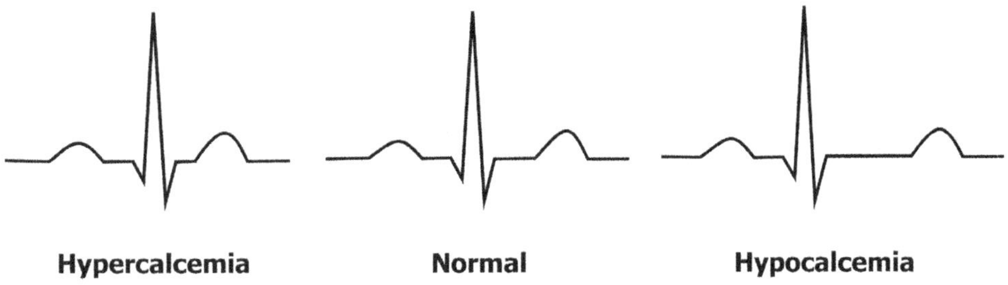

Figure 1.19: Changes in QT interval in moderate hypercalcemia and hypocalcemia.

If hypercalcemia becomes severe (>3.4 mmol/L) then Osborne waves (or J-waves) may be seen—an extra wave seen at the J-point of the ECG (the R-ST junction). The pathophysiology of the J-wave (figure 1.20) is poorly understood, but it is likely caused by an early repolarization of the epicardium—think of it as a chunk of early T-wave. (The other common cause of J-waves is hypothermia.) During hypocalcemia (<2.2 mmol/L) the opposite changes are seen in the ECG—the QT interval is prolonged, primarily due to a lengthened ST segment (figure 1.19).

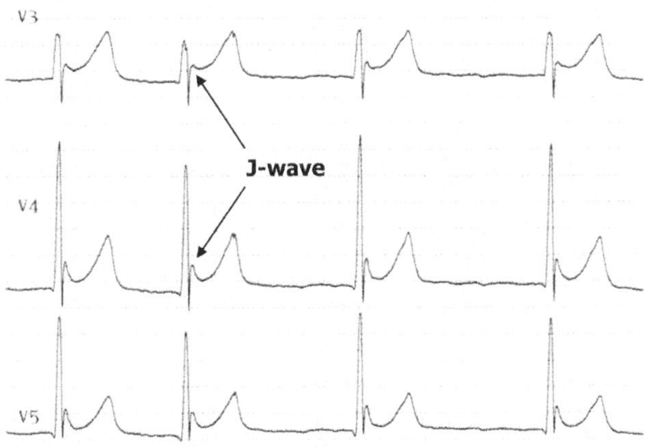

Figure 1.20: J-waves arise during hypothermia but can also be caused by hypercalcemia.

Hypercalcemia summary	Hypocalcemia Summary
Reduced ST and QT intervals	Prolonged ST and QT intervals
J-waves in severe hypercalcemia	

Table 1.16: Hyper- and hypocalcemia summary.

Hyper- and Hypokalemia

The pathophysiology is not as simple as changes in extracellular K^+ changing the electrochemical gradient for K^+. Because of potassium's role in maintaining the resting membrane potential, shifts in extracellular potassium can also influence the activity of Na^+ and Ca^{++} channels.

Your intuition may lead you to think that hypokalemia (<2.7 mmol/L) would increase K^+ conductances because there is a greater gradient from inside to outside the cell, but that is not the case. Instead hypokalemia suppresses K^+ channel conductances by destabilizing K^+ channels. With low K^+ conductance, the ECG changes reflect problems with repolarization. The T-wave is flattened and can be inverted, and a prominent U-wave may be seen in the precordial leads (figure 1.21). ST depression may also be apparent.

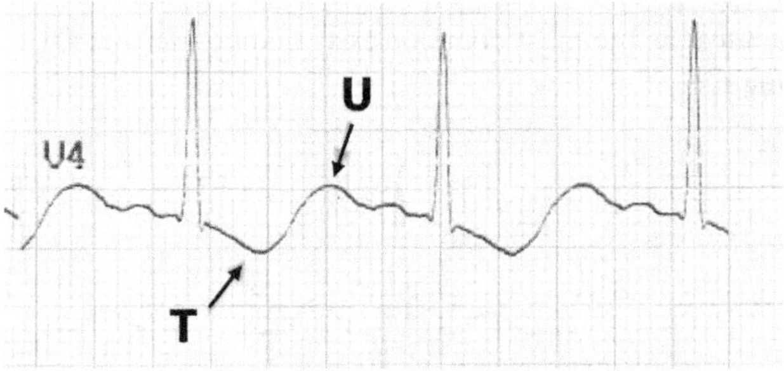

Figure 1.21: A prominent U-wave and inverted T-wave associated with hypokalemia.

As hypokalemia also inhibits Na^+-K^+ ATPase, Na^+ accumulates inside the cell. This in turn leads to an accumulation of Ca^{++} because of a subsequent failure of the Na^+-Ca^{++} exchanger. Extended presence of these two positive ions inside the myocyte prolongs the action potential and may manifest as an increased width and amplitude of the P-wave.

As hypokalemia worsens, the problems with K^+ conductance and repolarization increase, and the myocardium becomes susceptible to early after-depolarization (EAD) arrhythmias.

As K^+ is retained in the myocyte (due to the poor K^+ conductance) and elevated intracellular Na^+ and Ca^{++} results in the myocyte being more capable of depolarizing again. Because these after-depolarizations (figure 1.22) may not be uniform across the whole myocardium, an arrhythmia can be established. Potential arrhythmias include life-threatening forms, such as VT, VF, or torsades de pointes.

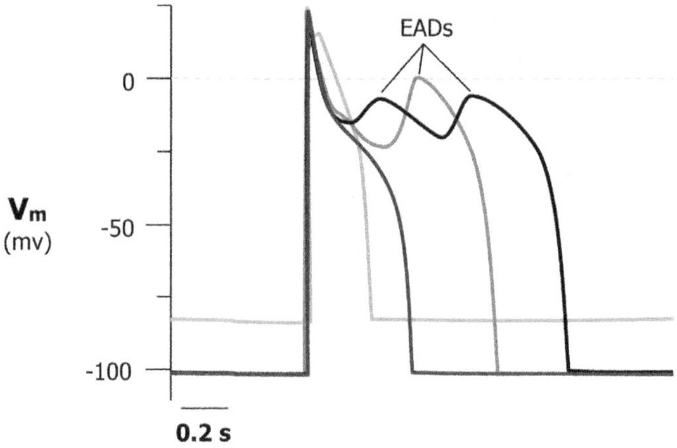

Figure 1.22: Early after-depolarizations occurring in a cardiac action potential due to poor K+ conductance in hypokalemia.

Hyperkalaemia produces different changes in myocardial excitability depending on the degree of excess potassium. Again the changes in excitability do not necessarily follow an intuitive logic of the change in the electrochemical gradient of K+. Mild hyperkalemia (5.5–6.5 mEq/L) causes peaked T-waves (figure 1.23)—the first sign of raised extracellular potassium. The excess potassium allosterically interferes with K^+ channels and, inverse to hypokalemia, causes an increase in K^+ conductance (despite the lower transmembrane gradient).

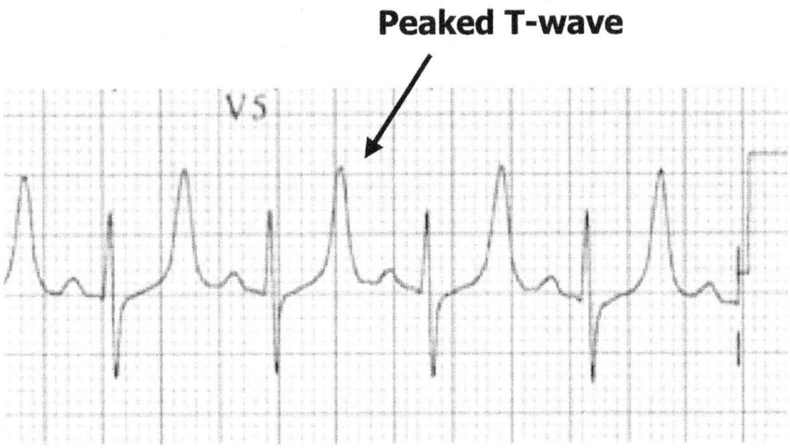

Figure 1.23: Peaked T-waves with mild hyperkalemia.

Moderate hyperkalemia (5.5–6.5 mEq/L) raises the membrane potential closer to the threshold of voltage-gated Na^+ channels (-70 mV) and voltage-gated Ca^{++}channels. Consequently these channels are more likely to fire and cause depolarization, hence the myocardium is initially more excitable. However, this persistent depolarization leaves the slow deactivation (h) gates on Na^+ channels closed for longer, and the ECG manifestations soon reflect a decreased excitability. The P-wave is longer but has low amplitude (and may eventually disappear), the QT interval is prolonged, and there is a decreased R-wave amplitude (figure 1.24). In simpler terms, the overstimulation of Na^+ channels causes them to "lock up."

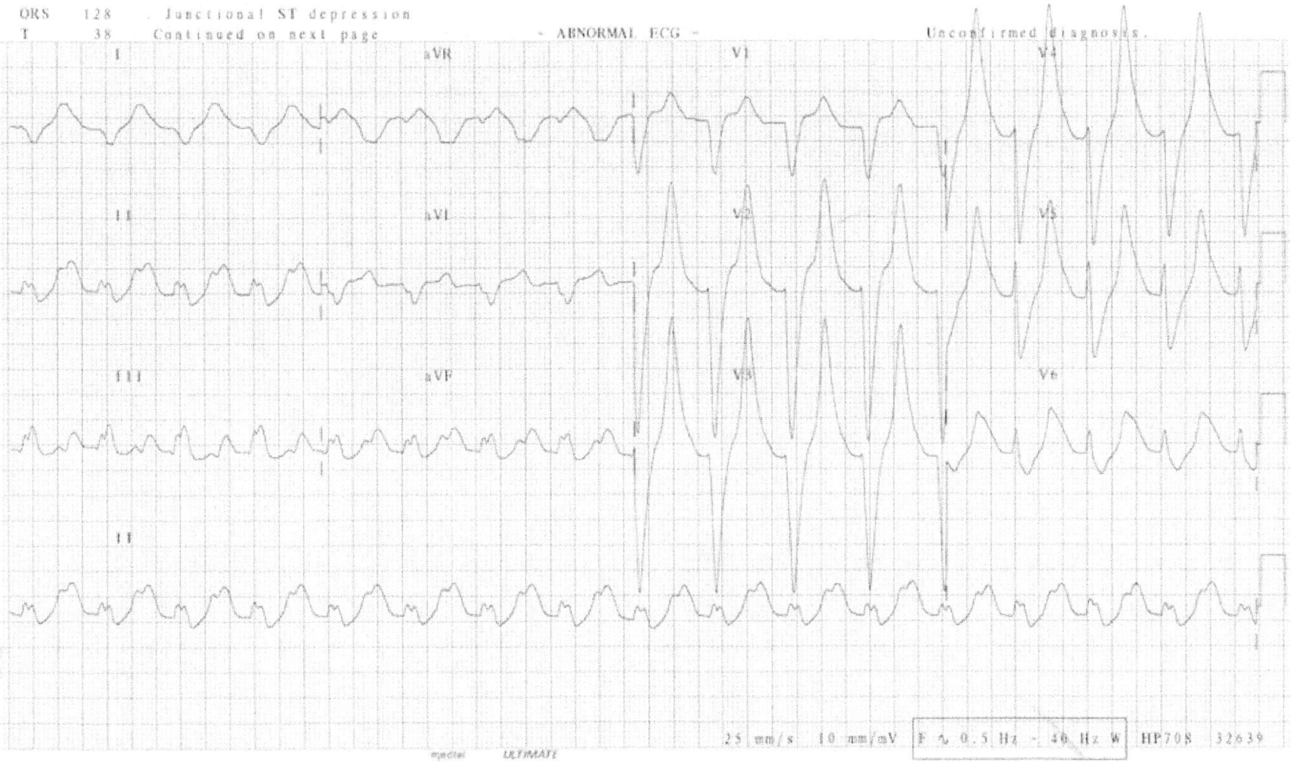

Figure 1.24: Big T, and little p and r of moderate hyperkalemia.

Severe hyperkalemia (>7.0 mEq/L) sees a worsening of the unresponsiveness of the myocardium, and the SA node rhythm is slowed, producing sinus bradycardia until there is no P-wave. Conductive issues arise, and a high-grade atrioventricular block is likely, allowing ventricular pacemakers to take over, but the ventricular myocardium is also unresponsive, so the QRS complex becomes broad and sine wave–like on the ECG (figure 1.25); this is a preterminal rhythm. At this point cardiovascular collapse and death are imminent, often through a VF finale.

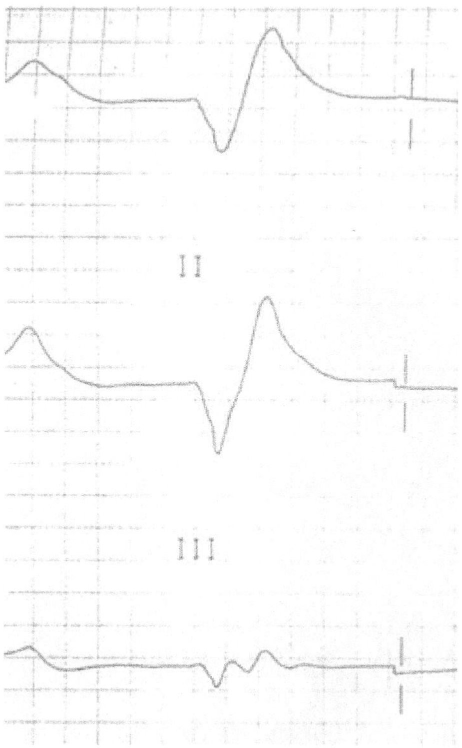

Figure 1.25: Preterminal ECG of severe hyperkalemia.

Hypokalemia summary	**Hyperkalemia summary**
Flattened or inverted T-wave	Mild: Peaked T-waves
Increased P-wave amplitude	Moderate: Long P-wave, prolonged QT interval, decreased amplitude R-wave
Induced arrhythmias in severe hypokalemia	Severe: Loss of P-wave, ventricular sine wave action potential

Table 1.17: Hypo- and hyperkalemia summary.

References, resources, and further reading

Text

Burns, Ed, and Robert Buttner. *Hypercalcaemia.* Lift in the Fast Lane, 2021. https://litfl.com/hypercalcaemia-ecg-library/, CC BY 4.0.

Burns, Ed, and Robert Buttner. *Hypocalcaemia.* Life in the Fast Lane, 2021. https://litfl.com/hypocalcaemia-ecg-library/, CC BY 4.0.

Buttner, Robert, and Ed Burns. *Hyperkalaemia.* Life in the Fast Lane. https://litfl.com/hyperkalaemia-ecg-library/, CC BY 4.0.

Buttner, Robert, and Ed Burns. *Hypokalaemia.* Life in the Fast Lane, 2021. https://litfl.com/hypokalaemia-ecg-library/, CC BY 4.0.

Chhabra, Lovely, Amandeep Goyal, and Michael D. Benham. *Wolff Parkinson White Syndrome.* Treasure Island, FL: StatPearls Publishing, 2022. https://www.ncbi.nlm.nih.gov/books/NBK554437/, CC BY 4.0.

Custer, Adam M., Varun S. Yelamanchili, and Sarah L. Lappin. *Multifocal Atrial Tachycardia.* Treasure Island, FL: StatPearls Publishing, 2022. https://www.ncbi.nlm.nih.gov/books/NBK459152/, CC BY 4.0.

Farzam, Khashayar, and John R. Richards. *Premature Ventricular Contraction.* Treasure Island, FL: StatPearls Publishing, 2022. https://www.ncbi.nlm.nih.gov/books/NBK532991/, CC BY 4.0.

Foth, Christopher, Manesh Kumar Gangwani, and Heidi Alvey. *Ventricular Tachycardia.* Treasure Island, FL: StatPearls Publishing, 2022. https://www.ncbi.nlm.nih.gov/books/NBK532954/, CC BY 4.0.

Hafeez, Yamama, and Shamai A. Grossman. *Sinus Bradycardia.* Treasure Island, FL: StatPearls Publishing, 2022. https://www.ncbi.nlm.nih.gov/books/NBK493201/, CC BY 4.0.

Harkness, Weston T., and Mary Hicks. *Right Bundle Branch Block.* Treasure Island, FL: StatPearls Publishing, 2022. https://www.ncbi.nlm.nih.gov/books/NBK507872/, CC BY 4.0.

Heaton, Joseph, and Srikanth Yandrapalli. *Premature Atrial Contractions.* Treasure Island, FL: StatPearls Publishing, 2022. https://www.ncbi.nlm.nih.gov/books/NBK559204/, CC BY 4.0.

Kashou, Anthony H., Amandeep Goyal, Tran Nguyen, and Lovely Chhabra. *Atrioventricular Block.* Treasure Island, FL: StatPearls Publishing, 2022. https://www.ncbi.nlm.nih.gov/books/NBK459147/, CC BY 4.0.

"Learn the Heart." Healio. https://www.healio.com/cardiology/learn-the-heart.

Ludhwani, Dipesh, Amandeep Goyal, and Mandar Jagtap. *Ventricular Fibrillation.* Treasure Island, FL: StatPearls Publishing, 2022. https://www.ncbi.nlm.nih.gov/books/NBK537120/, CC BY 4.0.

Nesheiwat, Zeid, Amandeep Goyal, and Mandar Jagtap. *Atrial Fibrillation.* Treasure Island, FL: StatPearls Publishing, 2022. https://www.ncbi.nlm.nih.gov/books/NBK526072/, CC BY 4.0.

Pipilas, Daniel C., Bruce A. Koplan, and Leonard S. Lilly. "The Electrocardiogram." In *Pathophysiology of Heart Disease: A Collaborative Project of Medical Students and Faculty*, 5e edited by Leonard S. Lilly, Chapter 4. Philadelphia: Lippincott Williams & Wilkins, a Wolters Kluwer Business, 2010.

Rodriguez Ziccardi, Mary, Amandeep Goyal, and Christopher V. Maani. *Atrial Flutter*. Treasure Island, FL: StatPearls Publishing, 2022. https://www.ncbi.nlm.nih.gov/books/NBK540985/, CC BY 4.0.

Scherbak, Dmitriy, and Gregory J. Hicks. *Left Bundle Branch Block*. Treasure Island, FL: StatPearls Publishing, 2022. https://www.ncbi.nlm.nih.gov/books/NBK482167/, CC BY 4.0.

Figures

Figure 1.1: Atrial fibrillation. Grey, Kindred. 2022. CC BY-NC-SA 4.0. Added Burns, Ed, and Robert Buttner. Example 2 (image cropped), *Atrial Fibrillation*. Life in the Fast Lane, 2021. https://litfl.com/atrial-fibrillation-ecg-library/, CC BY-NC-SA 4.0. https://archive.org/details/1.1_20220113

Figure 1.2: Comparison of atrial arrhythmias, including atrial fibrillation, atrial flutter, and multifocal atrial tachycardia (MAT). Grey, Kindred. 2022. CC BY-NC-SA 4.0. Added Burns, Ed, and Robert Buttner. Example 1 (image cropped), *Multifocal Atrial Tachycardia* (MAT). Life in the Fast Lane, 2021. https://litfl.com/multifocal-atrial-tachycardia-mat-ecg-library, CC BY-NC-SA 4.0. Added Burns, Ed, and Robert Buttner. Example 4 (image cropped), *Atrial Fibrillation* (image cropped). Life in the Fast Lane, 2021. https://litfl.com/atrial-fibrillation-ecg-library/, CC BY-NC-SA 4.0. Added Buttner, Robert, and Ed Burns. Example 3 (image cropped), *Atrial Flutter*. Life in the Fast Lane, 2021. https://litfl.com/atrial-flutter-ecg-library/, CC BY-NC-SA 4.0. https://archive.org/details/1.2_20220113

Figure 1.3: Atrial flutter. Burns, Ed, and Robert Buttner. Example 5 (image cropped), *Atrial Flutter*. Life in the Fast Lane, 2021. https://litfl.com/atrial-flutter-ecg-library/, CC BY-NC-SA 4.0.

Figure 1.4: Three distinct P-wave morphologies in a case of MAT. Burns, Ed, and Robert Buttner. Example 1 (image cropped), *Atrial Flutter*. Life in the Fast Lane, 2021. https://litfl.com/atrial-flutter-ecg-library/, CC BY-NC-SA 4.0.

Figure 1.5: Atrial bigeminy in PAC. Dawn. "ECG Basics: Sinus Rhythm with Atrial Bigeminy" (image cropped). ECG Guru, 2012. https://www.ecgguru.com/ecg/ecg-basics-sinus-rhythm-atrial-bigeminy, CC BY-NC-SA 4.0.

Figure 1.6: PVCs have a wider complex and are followed by a compensatory pause. Burns, Ed, and Robert Buttner. Multifocal PVCs Example (image cropped, scale and arrows removed, and new arrows added), *Premature Ventricular Complex* (PVC). Life in the Fast Lane, 2021. https://litfl.com/premature-ventricular-complex-pvc-ecg-library, CC BY-NC-SA 4.0.

Figure 1.7: Monomorphic and polymorphic VT. Grey, Kindred. 2022. CC BY-NC-SA 4.0. Added Buttner, Robert, and Ed Burns. Monomorphic VT Figure, *Ventricular Tachycardia—Monomorphic* VT. Life in the Fast Lane, 2021. https://litfl.com/ventricular-tachycardia-monomorphic-ecg-library, CC BY-NC-SA 4.0. Added Smith, Stephen W. Polymorphic VT Figure (second image, cropped), "Polymorphic Ventricular Tachycardia." Dr. Smith's ECG Blog, October 12, 2013. http://hqmeded-ecg.blogspot.com/2013/10/polymorphic-ventricular-tachycardia.html, CC BY-NC-SA 4.0. https://archive.org/details/1.7_20220113

Figure 1.8: Torsades de Pointes. Grey, Kindred. 2022. CC BY-NC-SA 4.0. Added Burns, Ed, and Robert Buttner. Torsades de Pointes Figure (image superimposed), *Polymorphic VT and Torsades de Pointes (TdP)*. Life in the Fast Lane, 2021. https://litfl.com/polymorphic-vt-and-torsades-de-pointes-tdp, CC BY-NC-SA 4.0. https://archive.org/details/1.8_20220113

Figure 1.9: Example of ventricular fibrillation with no recognizable P-waves or QRS complexes. Burns, Ed, and Robert Buttner. Example 2, *Ventricular Fibrillation* (VF). Life in the Fast Lane, 2021. https://litfl.com/ventricular-fibrillation-vf-ecg-library, CC BY-NC-SA 4.0.

Figure 1.10: Example of first-degree block with P-R interval >0.2 seconds. Larkin, John, and Robert Buttner. First Degree Heart Block Figure, *First Degree Heart Block*. Life in the Fast Lane, 2021. https://litfl.com/first-degree-heart-block-ecg-library, CC BY-NC-SA 4.0.

Figure 1.11: Mobitz I (second-degree block) with P-R intervals shown in seconds. Grey, Kindred. 2022. CC BY-NC-SA 4.0. Added Burns, Ed, and Robert Buttner. AV Block: 2nd Degree, Mobitz Type I Figure (image superimposed), *AV Block: 2nd Degree, Mobitz I (Wenckebach Phenomenon)*. Life in the Fast Lane, 2021. https://litfl.com/av-block-2nd-degree-mobitz-i-wenckebach-phenomenon, CC BY-NC-SA 4.0. https://archive.org/details/1.11_20220113

Figure 1.12: Mobitz II (second degree block) with arrows showing P waves. P-R interval is stable and ratio is 3:1. Grey, Kindred. 2022. CC BY-NC-SA 4.0. Added Burns, Ed, and Robert Buttner. Mobitz Type II Rhythm Strip Figure (image superimposed), *AV Block: 2nd Degree, Mobitz II (Hay Block)*. Life in the Fast Lane, 2021. https://litfl.com/av-block-2nd-degree-mobitz-ii-hay-block, CC BY-NC-SA 4.0. https://archive.org/details/1.12_20220113

Figure 1.13: Third-degree block with P-waves (black arrows) having an SA node rate of 100 bpm and the ventricles depolarizing (blue arrows) at 33 bpm. Larkin, John, and Robert Buttner. Complete Heart Block Figure, *AV Block: 3rd Degree (Complete Heart Block)*. Life in the Fast Lane, 2021. https://litfl.com/av-block-3rd-degree-complete-heart-block, CC BY-NC-SA 4.0.

Figure 1.14: Example of LBBB with defining features labeled. Grey, Kindred. 2022. CC BY-NC-SA 4.0. Added Buttner, Robert, and Ed Burns. Example 1 (image superimposed), *Left Bundle Branch Block (LBBB)*. Life in the Fast Lane, 2021. https://litfl.com/left-bundle-branch-block-lbbb-ecg-library, CC BY-NC-SA 4.0. https://archive.org/details/1.14_20220113

Figure 1.15: Changes in R-wave morphology as differences in left and right depolarization produce an M-shaped wave. Buttner, Robert, and Ed Burns. LBBB Figure (image cropped), *Left Bundle Branch Block (LBBB)*. Life in the Fast Lane, 2021. https://litfl.com/left-bundle-branch-block-lbbb-ecg-library, CC BY-NC-SA 4.0.

Figure 1.16: Typical RSR' pattern (upper) and slurred S (lower) of RBBB. Grey, Kindred. 2022. CC BY-NC-SA 4.0. Added Typical RSR' Pattern ('M'-Shaped) QRS in V1 Figure (image superimposed), *Right Bundle Branch Block (RBBB)*. Life in the Fast Lane, 2021. https://litfl.com/right-bundle-branch-block-rbbb-ecg-library, CC BY-NC-SA 4.0. Added Wide Slurred S Wave in Lead I Figure (image superimposed), *Right Bundle Branch Block (RBBB)*. Life in the Fast Lane, 2021. https://litfl.com/right-bundle-branch-block-rbbb-ecg-library, CC BY-NC-SA 4.0. https://archive.org/details/1.16_20220113

Figure 1.17: Schematics of normal WPW syndrome conductivity pathways. Grey, Kindred. 2022. CC BY 4.0. https://archive.org/details/1.17_20220113

Figure 1.18: Delta wave of WPW syndrome. Grey, Kindred. 2022. CC BY-NC-SA 4.0. Added Cadogan, Mike, and Robert Buttner. ECG Delta Wave 3 Figure (image superimposed), *Delta Wave*. Life in the Fast Lane, 2022. https://litfl.com/delta-wave-ecg-library, CC BY-NC-SA 4.0. https://archive.org/details/1.18_20220113

Figure 1.19: Changes in Q-T interval in moderate hypercalemia and hypocalcemia. Grey, Kindred. 2022. CC BY 4.0. https://archive.org/details/1.19_20220113

Figure 1.20: J-waves arising at the J-point during hypothermia but can also be caused by hypercalcemia. Grey, Kindred. 2022. CC BY-NC-SA 4.0. Added Example 3 (image superimposed), *Osborn Wave (J Wave)*. Life in the Fast Lane, 2022. https://litfl.com/osborn-wave-j-wave-ecg-library, CC BY-NC-SA 4.0. https://archive.org/details/1.20_20220113

Figure 1.21: A prominent U-wave and inverted T-wave associated with hypokalemia. Buttner, Robert, and Ed Burns. Hypokalaemia Figure (image letters edited), *Hypokalaemia.* Life in the Fast Lane, 2021. https://litfl.com/hypokalaemia-ecg-library, CC BY-NC-SA 4.0.

Figure 1.22: Early after-depolarizations occurring in a cardiac action potential due to poor K+ conductance in hypokalemia. Grey, Kindred. 2022. CC BY 4.0. https://archive.org/details/1.22_20220113

Figure 1.23: Peaked T-waves with mild hyperkalemia. Grey, Kindred. 2022. CC BY-NC-SA 4.0. Added Buttner, Robert, and Ed Burns. Example 2 (image superimposed), *Hyperkalaemia.* Life in the Fast Lane, 2021. https://litfl.com/hyperkalaemia-ecg-library, CC BY-NC-SA 4.0. https://archive.org/details/1.23_20220113

Figure 1.24: Big T, little p and r of moderate hyperkalemia. Cadogan, Mike. Figure 4, *Hyperkalaemia Clinical Case.* Life in the Fast Lane, 2020. https://litfl.com/hyperkalaemia-clinical-case, CC BY-NC-SA 4.0.

Figure 1.25: Preterminal ECG of severe hyperkalemia. Buttner, Robert, and Ed burns. Figure 6 (image cropped), *Hyperkalaemia.* Life in the Fast Lane, 2021. https://litfl.com/hyperkalaemia-ecg-library, CC BY-NC-SA 4.0.

2. Heart Failure

Learning Objectives

- Define systolic and diastolic heart failure.
- Define heart failure with reduced and preserved ejection fraction.
- Define the compensatory mechanisms activated during heart failure as beneficial or maladaptive.
- Describe the morphological and histological changes to the myocardium in response to heart failure.

While there are numerous pathological causes of heart failure (examples in table 2.1), let us look at how three basic forms of cardiac dysfunction can contribute to impaired cardiac output and congestion. The failing heart may have:

1. **Impaired contractility**: A decline in contractility is perhaps easiest to visualize; the pumping action of the heart is ineffective/reduced, and blood cannot be cleared from the chambers.
2. **An overwhelming afterload**: An increased afterload causes the heart to have to work harder to eject blood, and failure to do so leads to poor ejection fractions and cardiac output.
3. **Problems with ventricular filling**: Impaired ventricular filling during diastole means that the heart has a low preload, but because it cannot pump out what it does not receive, then cardiac output is lower.

For whichever reason the end effect of the failure is a decline in blood flow out of the heart, and consequently congestion on the way in.

Form of dysfunction	Example causes
Impaired contractility	- Myocardial infarction - Coronary atherosclerosis - Severe anemia - Cardiomyopathy - Arrhythmias - Congenital heart disease
Increased afterload	- Severe lung disease - Hypertension - Sleep apnea - Valvular disease
Impaired ventricular filling/relaxation	- Cardiomyopathy - Arrhythmias - Congenital heart disease - Valvular disease

Table 2.1: Changes in cardiac function in different disease states.

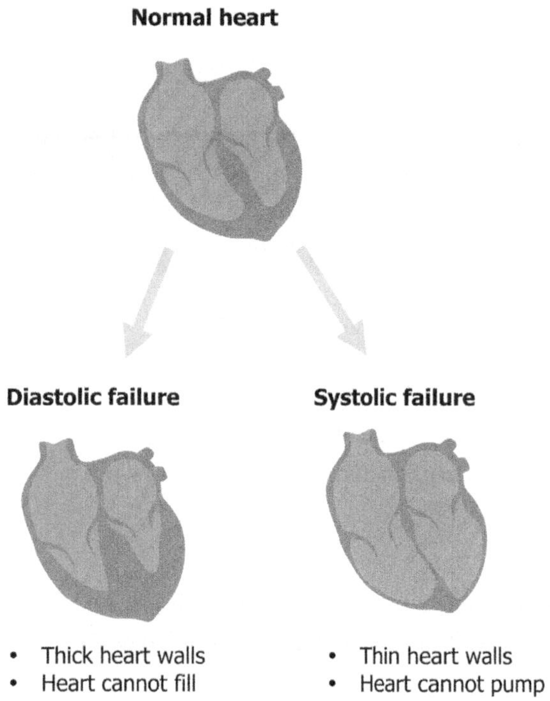

Figure 2.1: Overly simplified schema of heart failure. Systolic = cannot get the blood out; Diastolic = cannot get the blood in.

Impediments to emptying the heart during systole (i.e., a reduced contractility or increased afterload) were referred to as **systolic heart failure**. Similarly, problems with filling the ventricle during diastole were referred to as **diastolic heart failure** (figure 2.1).

In reality there is a great deal of overlap between these forms of heart failure, and elements of both can be present in the same patient. Similarly, as both forms result in congestion before the heart and reduced flow after it, they are hard to immediately distinguish. Consequently the type and degree of failure is now categorized by the effect on ejection fraction that can help distinguish the source of the problem.

$$\frac{\text{End-diastolic volume} - \text{End-systolic volume}}{\text{End-diastolic volume}}$$

Figure 2.2: Calculation for ejection fraction.

Heart Failure and Ejection Fraction

Let us quickly remind ourselves of what ejection fraction is. Ejection fraction is the proportion of blood volume that the left ventricle ejects in one beat. It is mathematically described as the starting volume (i.e., end-diastolic volume, EDV) minus the finishing volume (i.e., end-systolic volume, ESV) as a proportion of the starting volume (figure 2.2)—in simpler terms, what percentage of the ventricular blood volume was pushed out during a contraction.

Ejection Fraction in Systolic Failure

Let us first relate this to systolic failure by looking at what happens when the contractility of the myocardium is reduced. In systolic failure, there is a problem getting blood out of the heart, so the volume of blood coming out of the heart per beat (EDV-ESV) is reduced. However, the end diastolic volume will remain the same, or more likely rise. So our ejection fraction is reduced. Consequently, if you have a reduced ejection fraction you know you have a systolic failure. So to improve diagnosis, systolic failure is now referred to as heart failure with a reduced ejection fraction (HFREF).

Let us look at the pathophysiological consequences of HFREF. With a poor ejection fraction blood will begin to accumulate in the ventricle, and EDV will begins to rise and consequently so will the ventricular pressure. The raised pressure will impede venous return and promote venous congestion as blood struggles to enter the heart, and in the case of left ventricular failure the congestion will occur first in the left atrium and then in the pulmonary system (figure 2.3).

So systolic failure is referred to as HFREF, but what started as a problem emptying the heart has led to congestion and has produced a problem getting blood into the heart. Let us compare this with diastolic failure.

Ejection Fraction in Diastolic Failure

Remember that in diastolic failure there is a problem relaxing/filling the ventricle. Consequently EDV tends to be lower than normal, and this lower volume of blood in the chamber is relatively easy for the heart to expel. So proportionately, the ejection fraction can be maintained, even if the absolute stroke volume may be low. This is now classified as heart failure with a normal ejection fraction (HFNEF).

The pathophysiological consequences of HFNEF stem from the poor relaxation of the ventricle and/or ability to accept blood. When the ventricle is noncompliant during diastole (i.e., does not relax properly), it does not take much blood volume to enter the chamber before the ventricle pressure begins to rise. This rise in ventricular pressure opposes the entry of more blood, so it accumulates in the atrium. Atrial pressure rises and venous return is impeded, so blood becomes congested in the venous system.

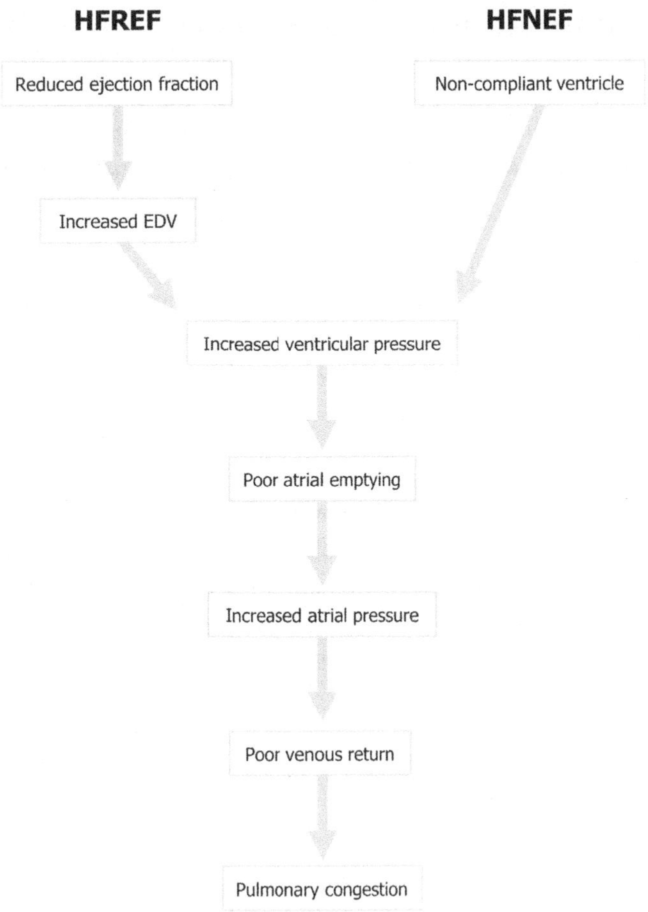

Figure 2.3: Pathophysiological sequence of left ventricular failure. Whether through lowered ejection fraction (HFREF, a.k.a. systolic failure) or through poor ventricular filling (heart failure with a normal ejection fraction, or HFNEF, a.k.a. diastolic failure), the end point of pulmonary congestion is the same.

If you compare this sequence of events in HFREF and HFNEF in figure 2.3 the end point is the same—congestion in the venous system, hence the difficulty in distinguishing "systolic" and "diastolic" failure and the need to measure ejection fraction and the newer categories of HFREF and HFNEF. In summary, HFREF starts with a problem getting blood out, that leads to a problem getting blood in, whereas HFNEF starts with a problem getting blood in that leads to a problem getting blood out. Both produce congestion, and both result in a diminished cardiac output.

Acute Responses to Reduced Cardiac Output in Heart Failure: Good or Bad?

Initial responses to the diminished cardiac output include the acute compensatory responses to low blood pressure, myocardial stretch, or changes in renal perfusion. Let us do a quick review.

The reduced cardiac output leads to a reduced arterial blood pressure, which, in combination with low volume exiting the heart, results in lower blood flow. With less blood exiting the heart, more remains in the chamber, particularly with systolic failure, so the myocardium is stretched. These three factors (pressure, flow, and myocardial stretch) elicit mechanical, neural, and hormone responses intended to correct the fall in pressure, resume flow, and clear the heart of congestion—but these responses are intended for a normal heart, not one undergoing failure.

First, the extended myocardium elicits the Frank-Starling mechanism to increase contractility, while the release of ANP and BNP induces sodium and fluid loss at the kidney. Conversely, reduced renal blood flow instigates the RAAS system to cause salt and fluid retention and vasoconstriction aided by the release of Endothelin-1 from the endothelium of flow-deprived vessels. Finally, the reduced arterial pressure prompts the baroreceptor reflex that increases sympathetic tone to increase rate and contractility, and antidiuretic hormone causes fluid retention. See the summary in figure 2.4.

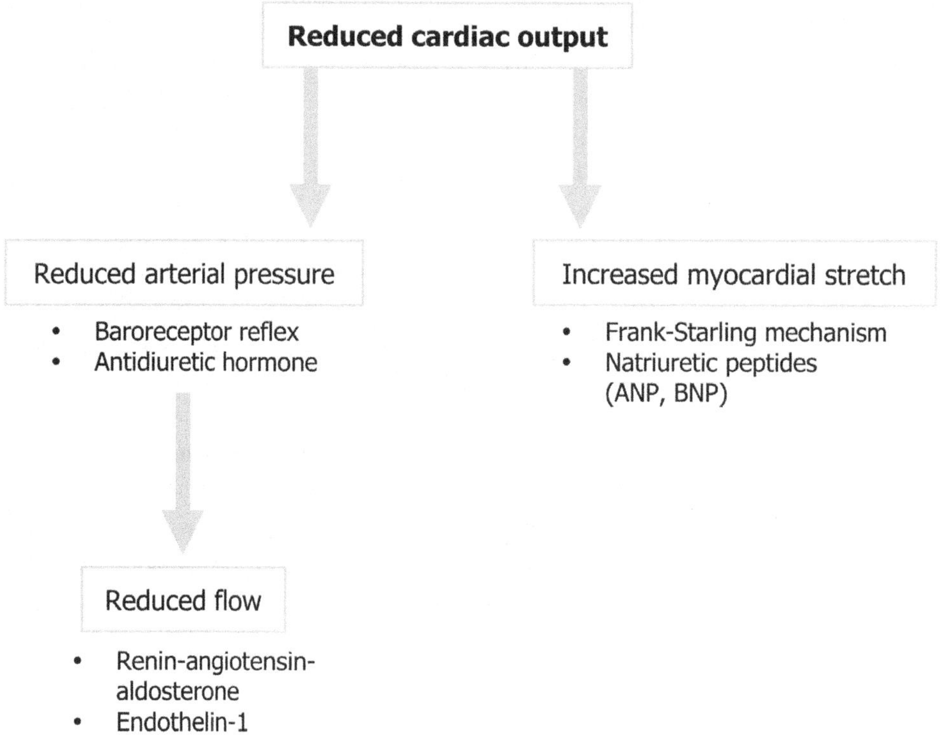

Figure 2.4: Compensatory responses to reduced cardiac output.

These compensatory effects are all attempts to improve cardiac output and blood pressure, but the failing heart is being forced to work harder against an increased afterload and move more volume. Consequently, but for the natriuretic peptides, these responses are maladaptive in the long term, and chronic changes to the heart are instigated.

Chronic Remodeling and Hypertrophy

The long-term structural changes begin with additional wall stress in the failing heart interacting with neurohormonal and cytokine alterations, but the wall stress seems to be an important instigator of hypertrophy and remodeling. Stress can be placed on the chamber walls in two major ways.

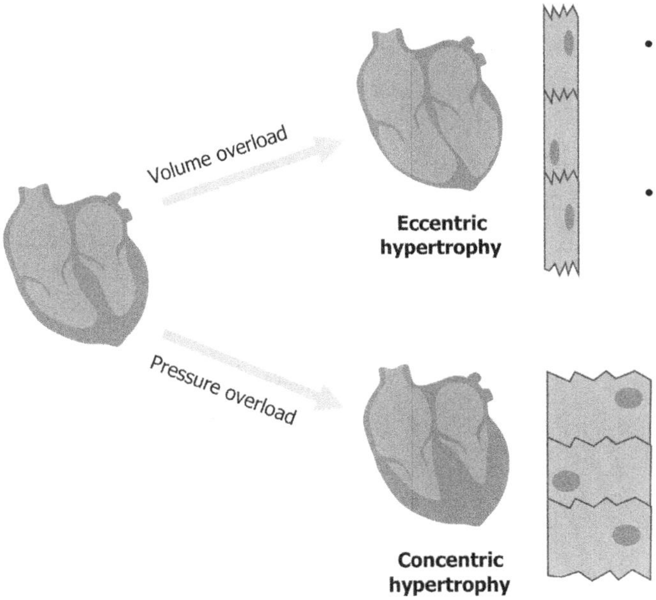

Figure 2.5: The effects of volume and pressure overload on the morphology of the heart and cardiac myocytes.

- **Volume overload** increases preload and consequently the chamber radius. Laplace's law states that this larger radius means the chamber wall must generate more tension to contain the same chamber pressure.
- **Pressure overload** creates higher demands to generate greater pressures to overcome an increased afterload. This requires additional wall tension and also leads to hypertrophy.

But the two forms of overload (volume and pressure) lead to different patterns of hypertrophy. In volume overload the myocytes add more sarcomeres in series, so they elongate and contribute to the dilation of the chamber while there is a proportional increase in wall thickness. This is referred to as eccentric hypertrophy (figure 2.5).

Pressure loading, on the other hand, leads to the synthesis of new sarcomeres that are formed in parallel to the old ones, causing an increase in wall thickness without any dilation of the chamber. This is referred to as concentric hypertrophy (figure 2.5).

These adaptations are accompanied by increased deposition of connective tissue that may have conductive or contractive ramifications. The difference in myocytic arrangement and presence of connective tissue is clear in the histological views of normal myocardium and myocardium chronically exposed to valvular disease in figure 2.6.

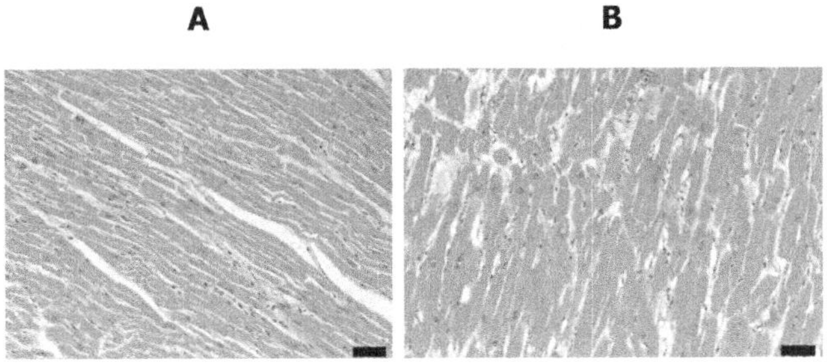

Figure 2.6: Normal myocardial (A) and myocardium exposed to valvular disease (B).

Myocytes may also be lost through either apoptosis or necrosis. As hypertrophy occurs the blood supply to the thickening wall becomes inadequate so infarction and consequent necrosis are more likely. Factors that promote myocyte apoptosis are all present during heart failure and include elevated catecholamines, Angiotensin II, inflammatory cytokines, and wall stress.

These same factors also disrupt gene expression in myocytes and cause intracellular deficits, including loss of Ca^{++} homeostasis and production of high-energy phosphates. While the mechanisms of these intracellular effects is still being heavily researched, the inability to control calcium or regulate high-energy phosphates obviously has implications of excitation-contraction coupling.

So while hypertrophy may seem a sensible response in the failing heart, the patterns and inflammation and stress-driven changes are eventually maladaptive and lead to a progressive decline in cardiac function.

Clinical Manifestations of Heart Failure

The clinical manifestations arise as fluid begins to move from the blood to the interstitium due to congestion (see summary in figure 2.7).

If the right heart fails, there is a rise in systemic venous pressure and peripheral edema arises. There may be abdominal discomfort as the liver becomes engorged and a loss of appetite or nausea as gastrointestinal edema arises. If the left heart fails, then the pulmonary circulation is exposed to the congestion and pulmonary edema arises.

Low cardiac output reduces renal filtration, so urine formation maybe impaired. Similarly cerebral blood flow may be compromised, causing dulled mental status.

Orthopnea arises when the patient lays down and venous return toward the failing left ventricle increases, compounding the pulmonary congestion. Patients often sleep propped up on pillows to elevate the heart and lungs. In severe cases the patient may only be able to sleep upright in a chair.

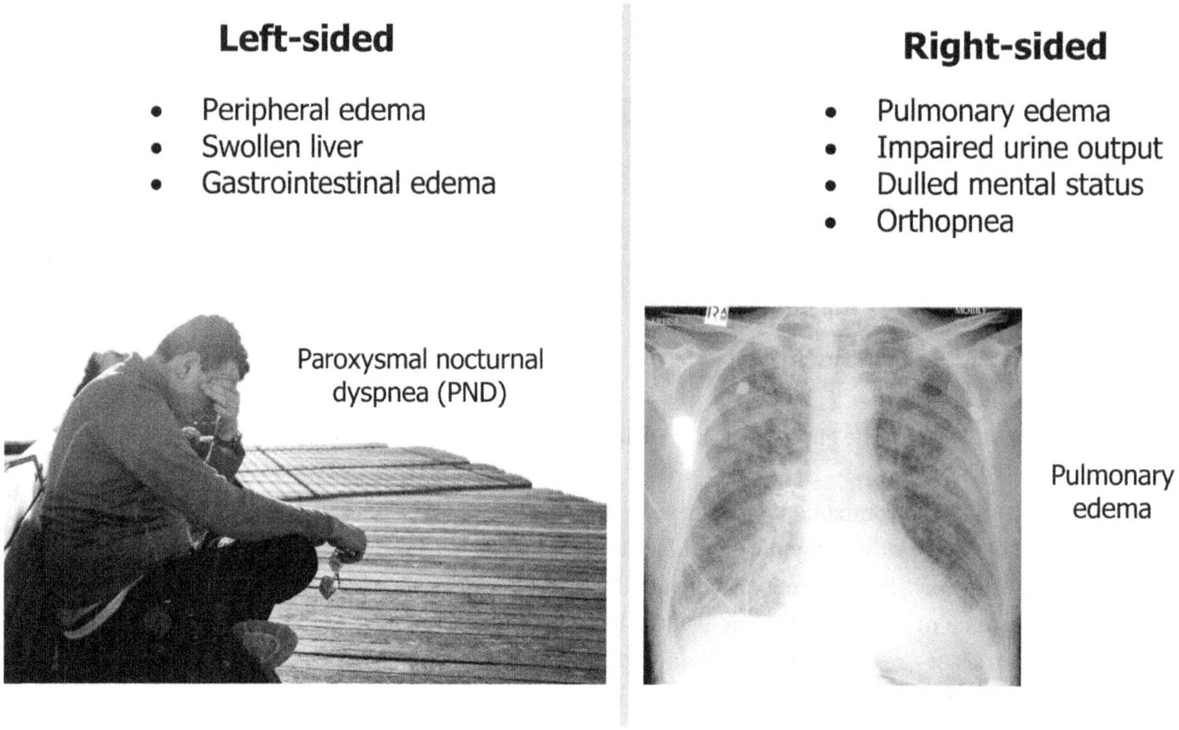

Figure 2.7: Consequences of right- and left-sided heart failure.

References, resources, and further reading

Text

Eberly, Lauren A., Eldrin F. Lewis, and Leonard S. Lilly. "Heart Failure." In *Pathophysiology of Heart Disease: A Collaborative Project of Medical Students and Faculty*, 5e, edited by Leonard S. Lilly, Chapter 9. Philadelphia: Lippincott Williams & Wilkins, a Wolters Kluwer Business, 2010.

Malik, Ahmad, Daniel Brito, Sarosh Vaqar, and Lovely Chhabra. *Congestive Heart Failure*. Treasure Island, FL: StatPearls Publishing, 2022. https://www.ncbi.nlm.nih.gov/books/NBK430873/, CC BY 4.0.

Figures

Figure 2.1: Overly simplified schema of heart failure. Systolic = can't get the blood out; Diastolic = can't get the blood in. Grey, Kindred. 2022. CC BY 4.0. https://archive.org/details/2.1_20220113

Figure 2.2: Calculation for ejection fraction. Grey, Kindred. 2022. CC BY 4.0. https://archive.org/details/2.2_20220113_202201

Figure 2.3: Pathophysiological sequence of left ventricular failure. Grey, Kindred. 2022. CC BY 4.0. https://archive.org/details/2.3_20220113

Figure 2.4: Compensatory responses to reduced cardiac output. Grey, Kindred. 2022. CC BY 4.0. https://archive.org/details/2.4_20220113

Figure 2.5: The effects of volume and pressure overload on the morphology of the heart and cardiac myocytes. Grey, Kindred. 2022. CC BY 4.0. https://archive.org/details/2.5_20220113

Figure 2.6: Normal myocardium (A) and myocardium exposed to valvular disease (B). Kakimoto, Yu, Chisa Okada, Noboru Kawabe, Ayumi Sasaki, Hideo Tsukamoto, Ryoko Nagao, and Motoki Osawa. "Myocardial Lipofuscin Accumulation in Ageing and Sudden Cardiac Death." *Scientific Reports* 9, no. 1 (2019). From Nature, CC BY 4.0.

Figure 2.7: Consequences of right- and left-sided heart failure. Grey, Kindred. 2022. CC BY-SA 3.0. Added Aguirre, Bruno. "Man Sitting on Bench beside Woman Photo." 2017, from Unsplash, CC BY-NC 4.0. Added Gaillard, Frank. "Pulmonary Oedema." 2011, from WikimediaCommons, CC BY-SA 3.0. https://archive.org/details/2.7-new

3. Hypertension

Learning Objectives

- Distinguish between essential and secondary hypertension.
- Describe the consequences of unmanaged hypertension.

Over seventy million Americans are hypertensive, and the Framingham study suggests that 90 percent of those over fifty-five years old will develop hypertension. But two-thirds of hypertensive patients are unaware of their condition so are exposed to the long-term effects.

The current guidelines (JNC 8, 2017) list the following pressures and categories to define hypertension:

- Normal (<120/80 mm Hg)
- Elevated (120–129/<80 mm Hg)
- Stage 1 hypertension (130–139/80–89 mm Hg)
- Stage 2 hypertension (≥140/90 mm Hg)

Essential Hypertension

Hypertension can be categorized as either **essential** or **secondary**. Secondary is much less common and a consequence of another condition (e.g., renal or endocrine disease). Essential hypertension (EH), despite being the prevalent form, is poorly understood but can be attributed to a problem with either cardiac output or peripheral resistance (i.e., the components of blood pressure regulation). Because multiple factors contribute to these components AND there is evidence of some genetic component to hypertension AND due to the contribution from environmental factors, essential hypertension can be considered a "description" rather than a "diagnosis." Primary abnormalities that may contribute to essential hypertension are shown in figure 3.1.

Genetic components of essential hypertension

No single loci has been identified as causing hypertension, but strong familial histories suggest polygenic causes (i.e., multiple loci are involved). Much attention has been paid to genes involved with enzymes and receptor production within the Renin-Angiotensin-Aldosterone (RAA) system because of its critical role in blood pressure control through sodium and volume regulation. Similarly genes involved with renal regulation of sodium have been studied. Our inability to demonstrate a genetic basis to hypertension is also consistent with significant environmental causes.

Systemic abnormalities and EH

Since Blood Pressure = Cardiac Output x Peripheral Resistance, it should be easy to imagine why aberrant rises in cardiac output (e.g., increased sympathetic tone) or peripheral resistance (e.g., low levels of vasodilators) would cause a rise in blood pressure (BP). Some of those aberrations of the acute BP control mechanisms are in figure 3.1, but this is clearly half the story as there are chronic control mechanisms that should surely compensation for loss of acute control. What this means is, for hypertension to be sustained, the kidney must be "in on the hypertension act." While the kidney itself can be responsible for volume-based hypertension (dysregulated renal blood flow, ion channels defects, etc.), there are deficits in renal control in hypertension. Renin levels are normal or high in 70 to 75 percent of EH patients—and of course they should be low as elevated BP should suppress renin secretion. So while this begins a chicken-and-egg scenario, for hypertension to be sustained, both acute and chronic control mechanisms must fail.

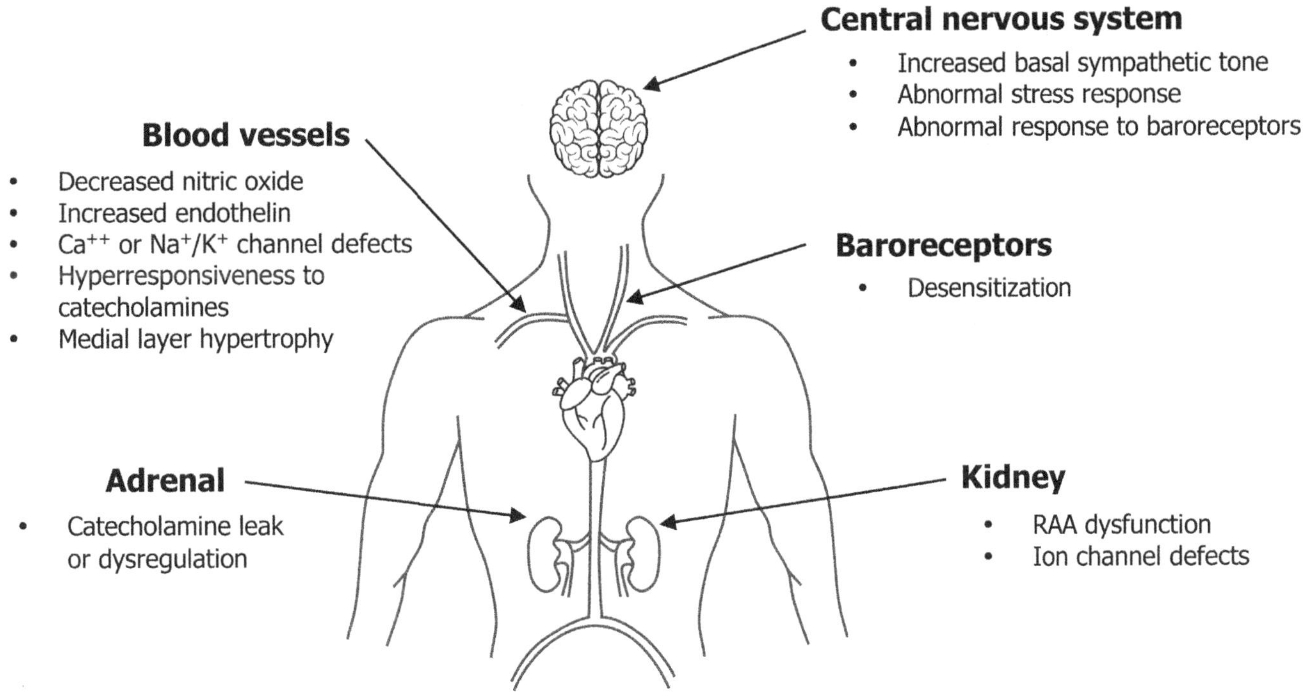

Figure 3.1: Potential sources of essential hypertension.

Diabetes, obesity, and EH

The linkage between diabetes and EH, and obesity and EH, appears strong and direct. Because insulin is a dietary-induced mediator of sympathetic activity, the elevated insulin levels in insulin-resistant diabetes can directly promote hypertension. Insulin can also lead to an increase in peripheral resistance via its mitogenic effect on vascular smooth muscle that causes hypertrophy in the medial vascular layers and a decrease in lumen size.

Obesity can also induce hypertension through release of angiotensinogen from more abundant adipocytes, thus providing more substrate for the RAA system. The increase in body mass is also accompanied by an increase in blood volume, and that blood may be more viscous as the large population of adipocytes release coagulative proteins, including prothrombin.

Secondary Hypertension

Although not as common, there are numerous causes of secondary hypertension. There are some distinguishing features that are clinically useful to distinguish it from EH. Your first heads-up is if the patient is younger and not in the typical range for EH (> fifty years old). Secondary hypertension also tends to be more severe, and BP can rise dramatically; EH does not have a rapid onset. While EH often comes with family history, secondary hypertension is more sporadic.

Suspicion of secondary hypertension can usually be confirmed by urinalysis that reveals the underlying issue (see table 3.1 for some common causes and cues for diagnosis). Disturbances in electrolytes and creatinine accompany the renal and mineralocorticoid-based diseases. Pheochromocytoma is rare and accounts for 0.2 percent of secondary hypertension cases (however, it is much more common in exam questions than it is in the clinic!).

Drugs that disrupt the angiotensinogen pathways (e.g., estrogens), are sympathomimetic (e.g., over-the-counter cold remedies), or promote sodium and water retention (e.g., NSAIDS) can all produce secondary hypertension.

Primary disorder	**Clinical cues**
Chronic renal disease	- Increased creatinine - Abnormal urinalysis
Primary aldosteronism	- Decreased serum potassium
Renovascular	- Abdominal bruit - Sudden onset - Decreased serum potassium
Pheochromocytoma	- Palpitations, diaphoresis, headache, weight loss - Episodic hypertension
Coarctation of the aorta	- Blood pressure in arms > legs - Blood pressure in right arm > left arm - Midsystolic click
Cushing syndrome	- Central obesity - Hirsutism

Consequences of Hypertension

As most hypertensive patients are asymptomatic, the condition can be left unmanaged and allowed to produce significant chronic effects. Most of these effects are caused by the extra work placed on the heart with the increased afterload and the damage to the interior of the vasculature.

The excess afterload can lead to systolic dysfunction and eventually heart failure with reduced ejection fraction (HFREF). In response to the excessive afterload the left ventricle can hypertrophy, causing a loss of compliance diastolic dysfunction and eventually heart failure with normal ejection fraction (HFNEF). The increased workload and muscle mass also increase the myocardial oxygen demand. This increase in demand often occurs at the same time that blood supply is diminished by concurrent atherosclerosis that is accelerated by the hypertension-induced arterial damage. Consequently, with high demand and low supply, the patient is prone to ischemia and myocardial infarction.

The arterial damage will also promote thrombosis and atheroemboli, so risk of embolic stroke is raised. Risk of hemorrhagic stroke is also increased as the vessel ways become weak. The large vessels are also at risk of being unable to counteract raised pressure (remember Laplace's law?), so aortic aneurysm and dissection can also occur.

High pressures entering the renal circulation can lead to nephrosclerosis. As renal function declines, a vicious cycle forms with renal failure exacerbating hypertension that exacerbates renal failure.

The retinal circulation provides a direct window into the state of the vasculature. Rapid onset and severe hypertension may burst small retinal vessels and produce local infarctions. In more chronic cases, arterial narrowing and medial hypertrophy of the retinal vessel can be seen. As the chronic hypertension worsens, arterial sclerosis is evident. While these chronic effects may not produce functional issues, they are at least an accessible indicator of the vascular status. The consequences of hypertension are summarized in figure 3.2.

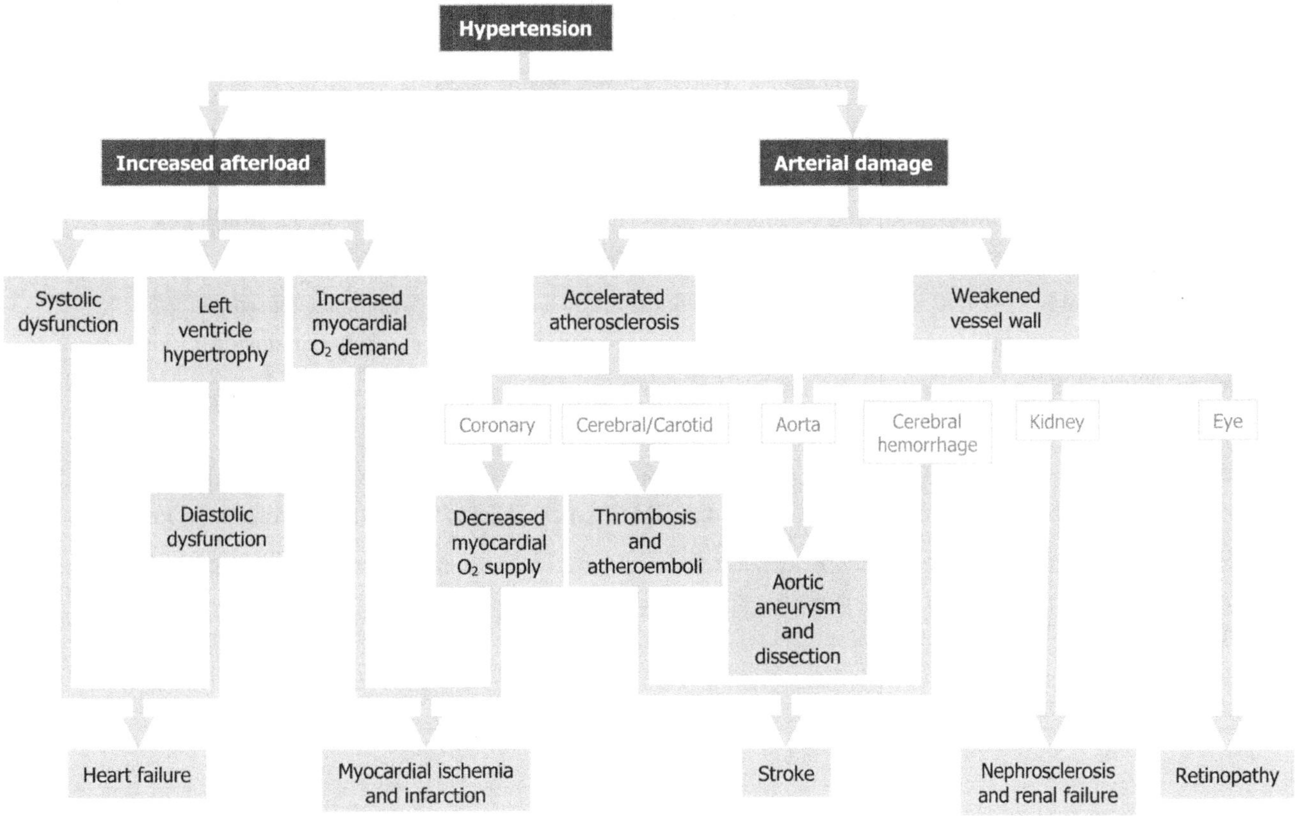

Figure 3.2: Consequences of hypertension.

Hypertensive Crisis

Most commonly caused by a hemodynamic insult overlaid on chronic hypertension, a hypertensive crisis is a severe elevation of blood pressure that can become life threatening through raising intracranial pressure. The rise in intracranial pressure produces severe headache, blurred vision, confusion, or even coma and is referred to as hypertensive encephalopathy. Funduscopy reveals retinal hemorrhages, exudates, and sometimes papilledema. The massive afterload on the left ventricle can precipitate angina. Therapy must be rapid to prevent permanent vascular consequences, and if administered in time the acute changes are usually reversed. However, the underlying cause of the crisis (usually renal failure) will persist.

References, resources, and further reading

Text

Brown, Jenifer M., Gordon H. Williams, and Leonard S. Lilly. "Hypertension." In *Pathophysiology of Heart Disease: A Collaborative Project of Medical Students and Faculty*, 5e edited by Leonard S. Lilly, Chapter 13. Philadelphia: Lippincott Williams & Wilkins, a Wolters Kluwer Business, 2010.

Hajar, Rachel. "Framingham Contribution to Cardiovascular Disease." *Heart Views* 17, no. 2 (April–June 2016): 78–81. https://www.ncbi.nlm.nih.gov/pmc/articles/PMC4966216.

Iqbal, Arshad Muhammad, and Syed F. Jaml. *Essential Hypertension*. Treasure Island, FL: StatPearls Publishing, 2022. https://www.ncbi.nlm.nih.gov/books/NBK539859/, CC BY 4.0.

Page, Michael R. "The JNC 8 Hypertension Guidelines: An In-Depth Guide." *Evidence-Based Diabetes Management* 20, no. SP1 (January 2014). https://www.ajmc.com/view/the-jnc-8-hypertension-guidelines-an-in-depth-guide.

Figures

Figure 3.1: Potential sources of essential hypertension. Grey, Kindred. 2022. CC BY 4.0. Added Amethyst Studio. "Heart." 2019, from Noun Project, CC BY 4.0. Added Knicky, Nicky. "Brain." 2015, from Noun Project, CC BY 4.0. https://archive.org/details/3.1_20220113.

Figure 3.2: Consequences of hypertension. Grey, Kindred. 2022. CC BY 4.0. https://archive.org/details/3.3_20220113

4. Valvular Disease

Learning Objectives

- Describe the major causes of valvular incompetence or stenosis.

In basic terms, normal valves maintain normal direction of blood flow through the heart's chambers. If they do not close properly they can allow backflow (regurgitation). If the valve does not fully open or is narrowed (stenosed), then the raised resistance impedes blood movement on its normal route and extra propulsive force must be applied by the myocardium. The clinical manifestations of cardiac valve disease vary depending on the valve involved, the form of dysfunction, and the severity and rate of onset of that dysfunction.

Abnormalities of valvular structure and/or function can either be congenital or acquired. Acquired valvular disease is by far the most common and is most prevalent in the elderly. The high blood flow and pressures that valves are exposed to make them particularly susceptible to other risk factors that promote valvular damage (see table 4.1). Congenital valvular defects arise from disrupted heart development, about 50 percent of which involve the valves. The impact of congenital defects has diminished with the advent of advanced detection techniques. What we will spend time on in this chapter is the main instigating factors and pathologies that result in acquired valvular defects.

Risk factors
Age
Gender
Tobacco use
Hypercholesterolemia
Rheumatic heart disease
Hypertension
Type II diabetes

Table 4.1: Risk factors for acquired valvular damage.

Pathophysiology of Valvular Disease

The constant stress of facing high flow and pressure over thirty to forty million cardiac contractions a year is not without its consequences, and the most common valvular disorder is calcification that comes with "wear-and-tear" and aging. The presence of other factors such as hyperlipidemia, hypertension, and inflammation accelerate this process and promote the deposition of hydroxyapatite (a form of calcium phosphate), and the valve structure contains cells that resemble osteoblasts (figure 4.1).

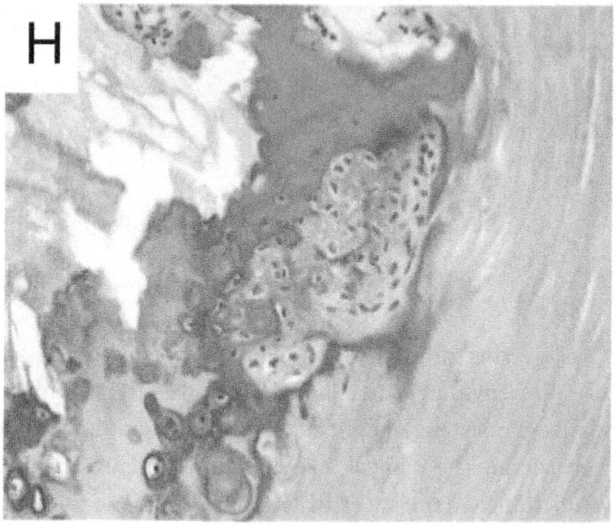

Figure 4.1: Histological view of the ossification of valve tissue with osteoblast-like cells clustered in the center of the field of view. These cells are responsible for the calcification and consequent stiffening of the valve leaflet.

As they face the most pressure, the aortic and mitral valves are more prone to calcification. The most common pattern of calcification in the aortic valve is mounded masses within the cusps of the valve (see table 4.2) that eventually fuse and stop the valve from opening fully. Calcification in the mitral valve tends to start in the fibrous annulus, which does not impact valvular function to the same extent, but in exceptional cases can cause regurgitation or stenosis, or even arrhythmias as calcium deposits impinge on the atrioventricular conduction system (see table 4.2).

Valve	Deposition of calcium	Gross path	Consequences
Aortic	Cusp	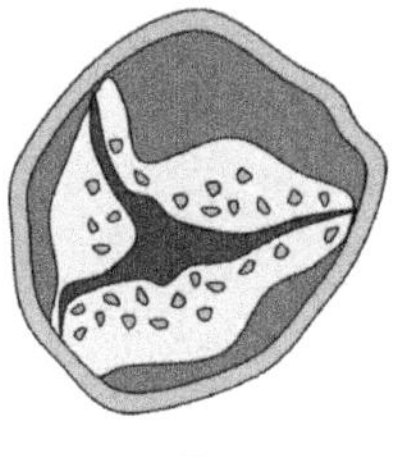	Stenosis
Mitral	Annulus	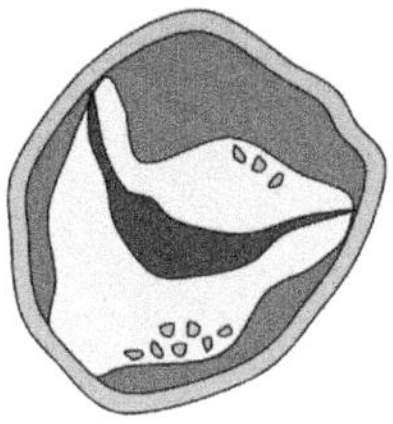	- Stenosis - Regurgitation - Arrhythmias

Table 4.2: Location of calcium deposits on aortic and mitral valves and their pathological consequences.

Mitral Valve Prolapse (MVP)

A prolapsed mitral valve is one where one or both leaflets have become floppy and capable of ballooning back into the left atrium during systole (figure 4.2). The condition is more common in women, affects 2–3 percent of adults in the United States, and can be a secondary effect of mitral valve regurgitation.

The causes of MVP are usually unidentified, but a few cases can be attributed to inherited connective tissue disorders such as Marfan syndrome. The prolapsed valve leaflet composition is enlarged and thickened with deposition of myxomatous material rich in proteoglycans, and a reduction in the structurally critical fibrosa layer where a higher prevalence of type III collagen (a more stretchy than structural form of collagen) is found.

The flapping valve structure can cause secondary fibrosis on the structures it strikes, such as the leaflet edges or the endocardium where the abnormally elongated cords rub. The agitation may also promote thrombus formation in the atrium.

The resultant floppy leaflet can be detected by a midsystolic click, and any associated incompetence may produce a late-systolic murmur (summary in figure 4.2). MVP is usually asymptomatic, but potential complications include:

- A propensity for endocardial infection,
- An increased risk of regurgitation and cord rupture,
- An increased stroke risk, and
- Higher incidence of arrhythmias.

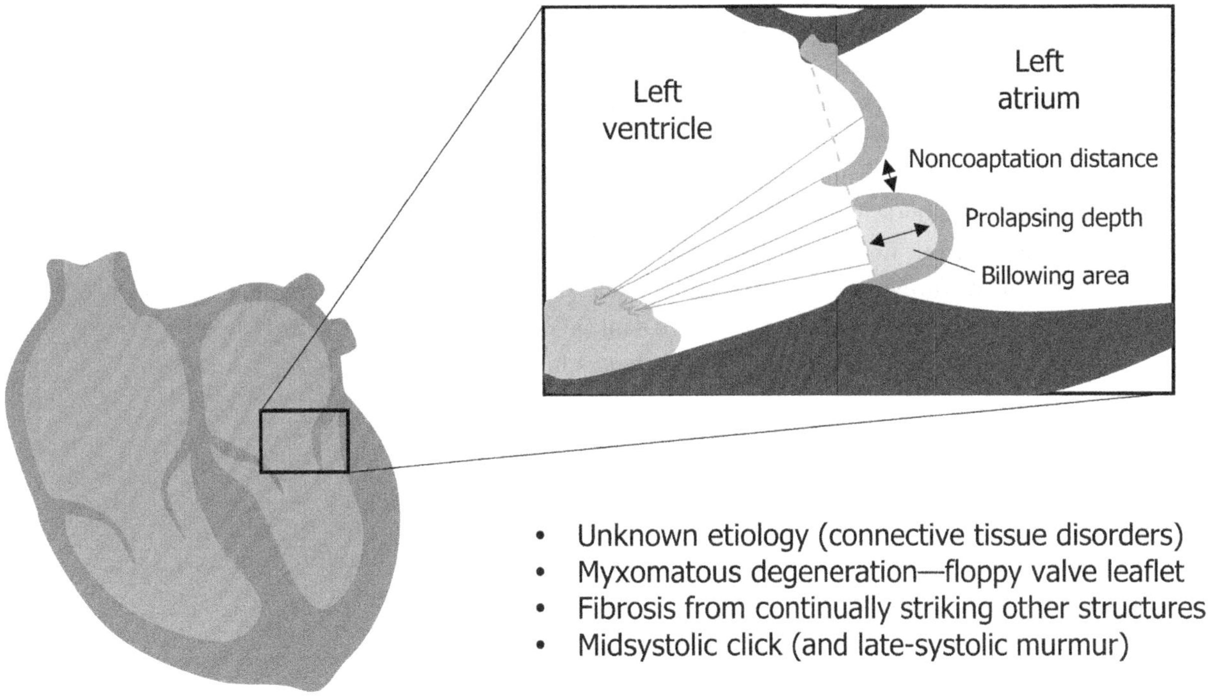

Figure 4.2: Mitral valve prolapse.

Rheumatic Heart Disease

Rheumatic heart disease (RHD) is virtually the only cause of mitral valve stenosis. It arises after a group A streptococcal infection that often originates in the upper airway and leads to rheumatic fever (a multisystem, immune-mediated disease). The incidence in developed countries is relatively low because of rapid diagnosis and treatment of the instigating pharyngitis, but in poor, crowed, urban areas RHD remains an important health issue.

The acute results of rheumatic fever occur days to weeks after the streptococcal infection, and while the initial pharyngeal infection may have cleared and the test results have become negative, the antibodies to the streptococcal enzymes (Streptolysin O and DNase B) can still be detected. The initial cardiac effects include carditis, pericardial rubs, tachycardia, and arrhythmias. However, the chronic effects may arise years or even decades later.

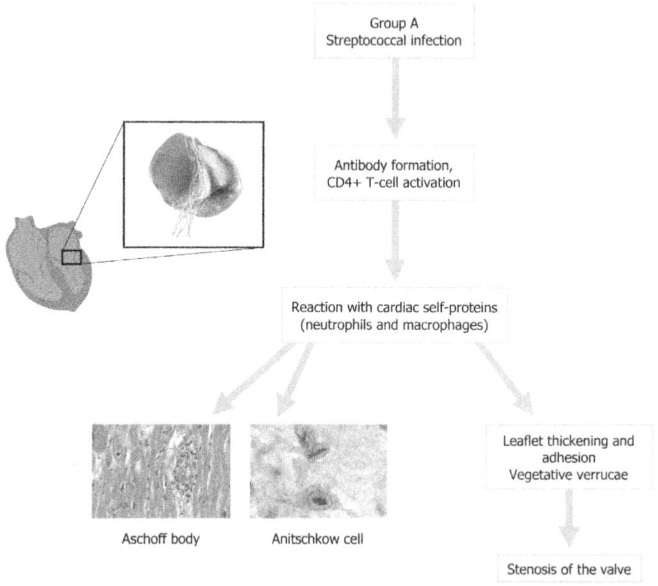

Figure 4.3: Pathophysiology of rheumatic heart disease.

The chronic effects involve an immune cross-reaction between the antibodies and CD4+ T-cells directed against the streptococcal M proteins and cardiac self-antigens. Antibody binding and T-cell activity toward the cardiac antigens activate complement and recruit neutrophils and macrophages toward the valve tissue. The damage they produce includes histologically distinct lesions called Aschoff bodies (figure 4.3), and plump activated macrophages called Anitschkow cells (or caterpillar cells) appear in the effected areas (figure 4.3). All layers of the myocardium can be effected, but the valves can show leaflet thickening and fusion as well as shortened, thickened cords. Vegetative verrucae are associated with the necrotic fibrinoid foci, making RHD one of the vegetative forms of valvular disease.

As the valve thickens it can become calcified as well, and the adhered leaflets produce a “fish-mouth” or “button hole” appearance that causes the valve to narrow. The damage is cumulative with the increased turbulence through a stenosed valve perpetuating the fibrotic process (see summary in figure 4.3).

Infective Endocarditis

Infective endocarditis (IE) is divided into acute and subacute forms, depending on the virulence of the causal pathogen. Acute IE is rapid in onset and involves highly destructive pathogens that cause necrosis and significant lesions that can lead to death in a matter of days. Subacute IE, alternatively, can deform the valves over weeks to months and generally involves a much less destructive pathogen.

Acute cases tend to involve healthy individuals and are responsible for 20 to 30 percent of cases, whereas the less virulent pathogens that cause subacute IE tend to need a foothold and only affect previously damaged or deformed valves.

Most incidence of IE start with fever, but it can also manifest as nonspecific fatigue, weight loss, or flu-like symptoms in older adults. The infection leads to vegetations on the valve that are the hallmark of IE (figure 4.4). These lesions contain fibrin, inflammatory cells, and bacteria.

The risk is twofold as the vegetations can:

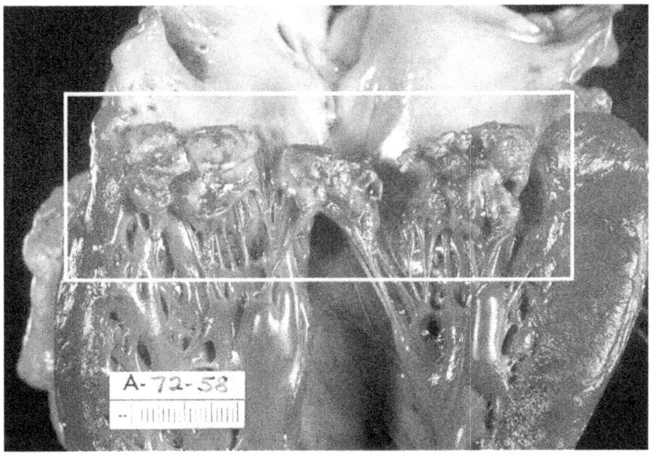

Figure 4.4: Vegetative lesions (in white box) associated with IE.

1. Disrupt valve function and form abscesses into the underlying myocardium, and
2. Embolize and carry the pathogens to a new septic infarcts or obstruct vasculature.

After a few weeks, complications arise that are the product of immune complex deposition or emboli. They can include glomerulonephritis as immune complexes become embedded in the glomerular basement membrane. Other later complications are now rare due to early detection and effective treatment but can include microthromboemboli that produce splinter or subungual lesions. Other hemorrhagic signs include Janeway lesions on the palms or soles, Osler nodes on the fingers, or Roth spots on the retina (figure 4.5).

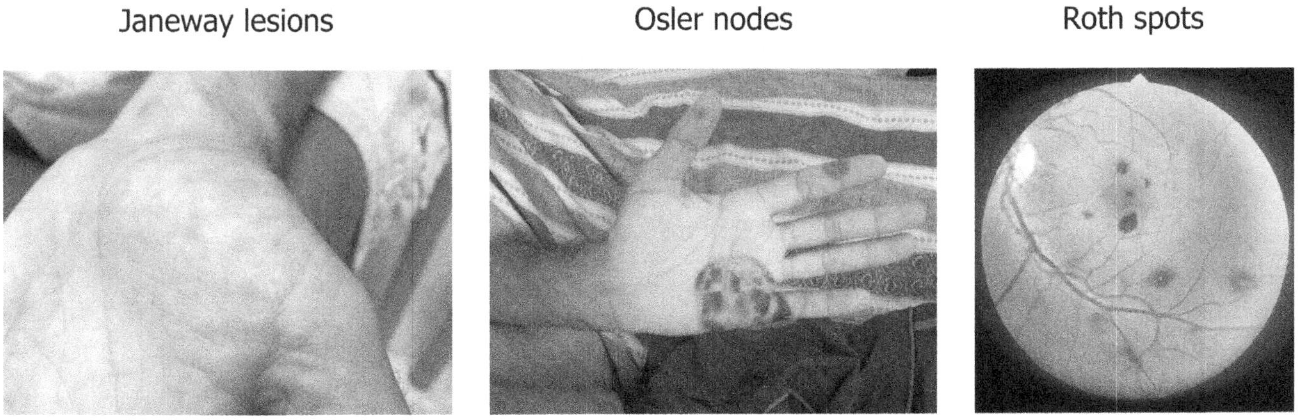

Figure 4.5: Signs of IE include Janeway lesions (left), Osler nodes (middle), and Roth spots (right).

Noninfective Vegetations

Some vegetations are sterile (i.e., occur in the absence of infection). There are two main examples of this—nonbacterial thrombotic endocarditis (NBTE) and the systemic lupus erythematosus (SLE).

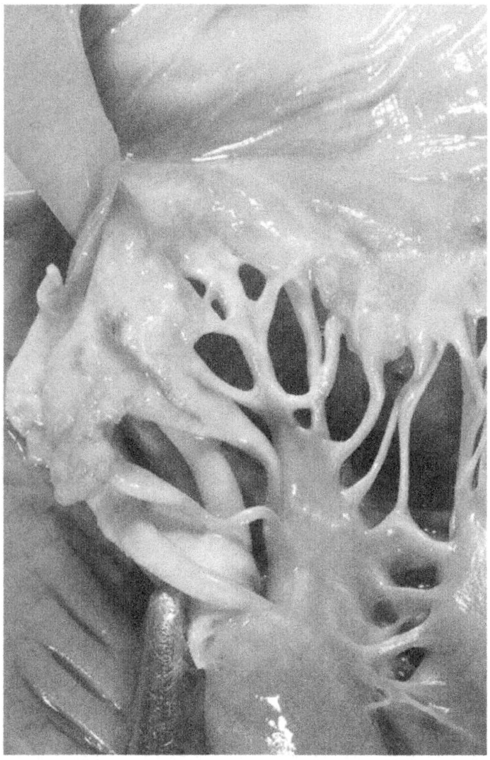

Figure 4.6: NBTE with small thrombi binding to valve leaflets.

Often coinciding with emboli in other sites, NBTE occurs in states of hypercoagulability, such as in cancer or sepsis. The small thrombi (1–5 mm) bind to the valve leaflets (figure 4.6), but do not illicit an inflammatory response nor are they invasive. Often the local consequences are trivial, but they can be the source of emboli that lead to infarcts in the brain, heart, or elsewhere.

In SLE, the vegetations are again sterile and small (1–4 mm) with a pink, wart-like appearance that are composed of eosinophilic material, granular material, and cellular debris. They tend to adhere to the undersurfaces of the atrioventricular valves, the valvular endocardium, and the cords (figure 4.7). Unlike NBTE, the vegetations can instigate complement and Fc-bearing cells that cause intense valvulitis. The end product of this is referred to as Libman Sacks disease.

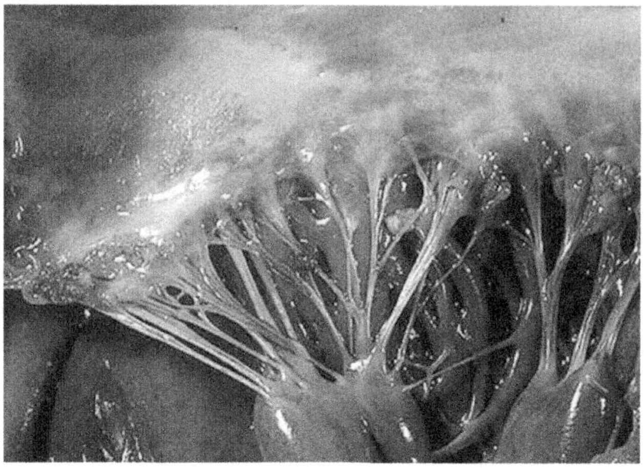

Figure 4.7: Small "wart-like vegetations" in the cords of a valve.

Carcinoid Heart Disease

Lastly, carcinoid heart disease is the cardiac manifestation of carcinoid syndrome. Carcinoid tumors are neuroendocrine tumors that usually arise in the gastrointestinal tract or lungs, and they secrete a number of mediators (figure 4.8) that can give rise to carcinoid heart disease.

The liver normally metabolizes these circulating mediators, but when the metastatic burden overwhelms hepatic clearance, the right heart is exposed to their effects (the left heart is somewhat protected by the degradation performed by the pulmonary circulation).

Of all these released mediators, serotonin is the most likely candidate for causing cardiac effects, although the mechanism is not clear. Once established, carcinoid lesions are distinctive white intimal thickenings (figure 4.8) composed of smooth muscle cells and collagen embedded in a mucopolysaccharide matrix. The most common manifestations are tricuspid insufficiency and pulmonary stenosis.

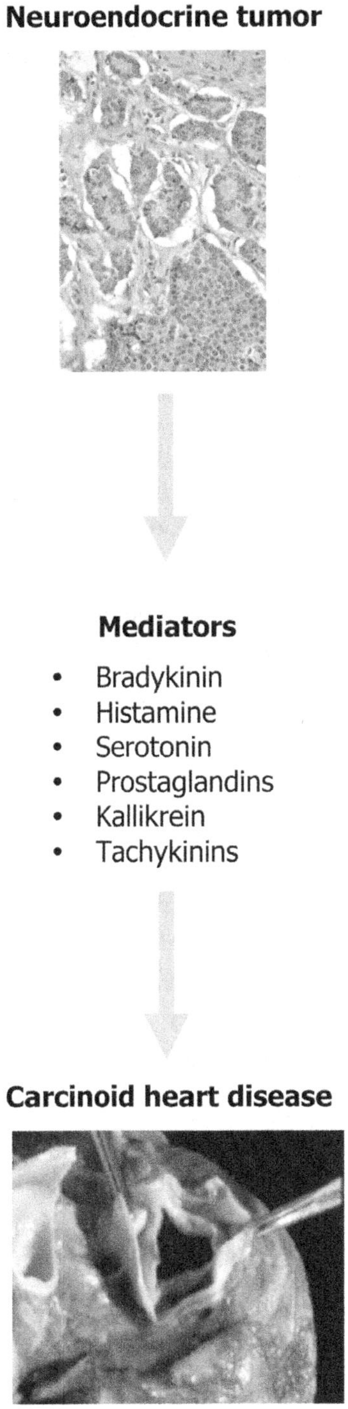

Figure 4.8: Release of inflammatory mediators from neuroendocrine tumors leading to carcinoid heart disease.

References, resources, and further reading

Text

Dass, Clarissa, and Arun Kanmanthareddy. *Rheumatic Heart Disease*. Treasure Island, FL: StatPearls Publishing, 2022. https://www.ncbi.nlm.nih.gov/books/NBK538286/, CC BY 4.0.

Douedi, Steven, and Hani Douedi. *Mitral Regurgitation*. Treasure Island, FL: StatPearls Publishing, 2022. https://www.ncbi.nlm.nih.gov/books/NBK553135/, CC BY 4.0.

Lopez, Diana M., Patrick T. O'Gara, and Leonard S. Lilly. "Valvular Heart Disease." In *Pathophysiology of Heart Disease: A Collaborative Project of Medical Students and Faculty*, 5e edited by Leonard S. Lilly, Chapter 8. Philadelphia: Lippincott Williams & Wilkins, a Wolters Kluwer Business, 2010.

Wenn, Peter, and Roman Zeltser. *Aortic Valve Disease*. Treasure Island, FL: StatPearls Publishing, 2022. https://www.ncbi.nlm.nih.gov/books/NBK542205/, CC BY 4.0.

Figures

Figure 4.1: Histological view of ossification of valve tissue with osteoblast-like cells. Torre, Matthew. Figure 1, "Osseous and Chondromatous Metaplasia in Calcific Aortic Valve Stenosis." *Cardiovascular Pathology* 25, no. 1 (January–February 2016): 18–24. From PubMed.gov, CC BY-NC-ND 4.0.

Table 4.1: Location of calcium deposits on aortic and mitral valves and their pathological consequences. Grey, Kindred. 2022. CC BY 4.0. https://archive.org/details/4.2a_20220113

Figure 4.2: Mitral valve prolapse. Grey, Kindred. 2022. CC BY 4.0. https://archive.org/details/4.3_20220113

Figure 4.3: Pathophysiology of rheumatic heart disease. Grey, Kindred. 2022. CC BY-SA 2.0. Added BruceBlaus. "Mitral Valve Prolapse." 2017, from WikimediaCommons, CC BY-SA 4.0. Added Nephron. "Rheumatic Heart Disease – 3b – Very High Mag." 2012, from WikimediaCommons, CC BY-SA 3.0. Added Uthman, Ed. "Anitschkow Myocytes in an Aschoff Body, Rheumatic Myocarditis." 2007, from WikimediaCommons, CC BY-SA 2.0. https://archive.org/details/4.4_20220113

Figure 4.4: Vegetative lesions (in white box) associated with IE. Centers for Disease Control and Prevention. "Haemophilus parainfluenzae Endocarditis PHIL 851 Lores." 1972, from WikimediaCommons, public domain.

Figure 4.5: Signs of IE include Janeway lesions (left), Osler nodes (middle) and Roth spots (right). Grey, Kindred. 2022. Added Community Eye Health. "Roth Spots and Retinal Haemorrhage." 1998, from Flickr, CC BY-NC 2.0. Added Galindo, Roberto J. "Osler Nodules Hand." 2010, from WikimediaCommons, CC BY-SA 4.0. Added Warfieldian. "Janeway Lesion." 2015, from WikimediaCommons, CC BY-SA 4.0. https://archive.org/details/4.6_20220113

Figure 4.6: NBTE with small thrombi binding to valve leaflets (arrowed). Mohsin, Sara. "Libman-Sacks Endocarditis." 2020, from WikiDoc, CC BY SA 3.0.

Figure 4.7: Small "wart-like vegetations" in the cords of a valve. Bouma, Wobbe, Iwan C. C. van der Horst, Theo J. Klinkenberg, and Inez J. Wijdh-den Hamer. "Mitral Valve Surgery for Mitral Regurgitation Caused by Libman-Sacks Endocarditis: A Report of Four Cases and a Systematic Review of the Literature." *Journal of Cardiothoracic Surgery* 5, no. 1 (March 2010): 13. DOI: 10.1186/1749-8090-5-13. *Reproduced in JCS with permission from Dr. S. Gonzalez. Copyright 2009, department of Pathology, Pontifical Catholic University of Chile, Santiago, Chile.* Used under fair use.

Figure 4.8: Release of inflammatory mediators from neuroendocrine tumors leading to carcinoid heart disease. Grey, Kindred. 2022. Added Feingold, K. R., B. Anawalt, A. Boyce, et al., eds. Figure 24, *Carcinoid Tumors*. South Dartmouth, MA: MDText.com, Inc., 2000–. From NCBI, CC BY-NC-ND 2.0. Used under fair use. Added Nephron. "Small Intestine Neuroendocrine Tumour High Mag." 2009, from WikimediaCommons, CC BY-SA 3.0.

5. Heart Sounds and Murmurs

Learning Objectives

- Describe the underlying events that produce the normal heart sounds, S1 to S4.
- Relate the timing and structure of a heart murmur to the underlying pathophysiology.

As unintrusive as the ECG is, listening to the heart is a cheap, quick, and informative clinical test. We will cover the basic structure, causes, and common pathologies of heart murmurs as a companion guide to clinical skills classes on auscultation of the chest. A good understanding of the cardiac cycle would be beneficial.

Heart Sounds

The first and second sounds (S1 and S2) are the fundamental heart sounds.

S1 occurs at the beginning of isovolumetric contraction. The ventricle is beginning to contract, so ventricular pressure quickly rises above atrial pressure and the atrioventricular (tricuspid and mitral) valves close, producing the S1 sound. The mitral valve normally closes slightly (0.04 seconds) before the tricuspid, causing S1 to be "split" (i.e., actually being two sounds, M1 and T1 (figure 5.1)), but the time gap is too short with a normal heart to be detectable with a stethoscope. The reasons for M1 preceding T1 are not clear, but may be due to the force generation of the left ventricle being slightly faster than that of the right ventricle. The splitting of S1 can be more pronounced and audible in the presence of a right bundle branch block (figure 5.1) that causes left ventricular contraction (and mitral valve closure) to markedly precede contraction of the right ventricle. Conversely, in the case of a left bundle branch block, the normal splitting of S1 may be absent (figure 5.1) as M1 is delayed and so occurs in synchrony with T1.

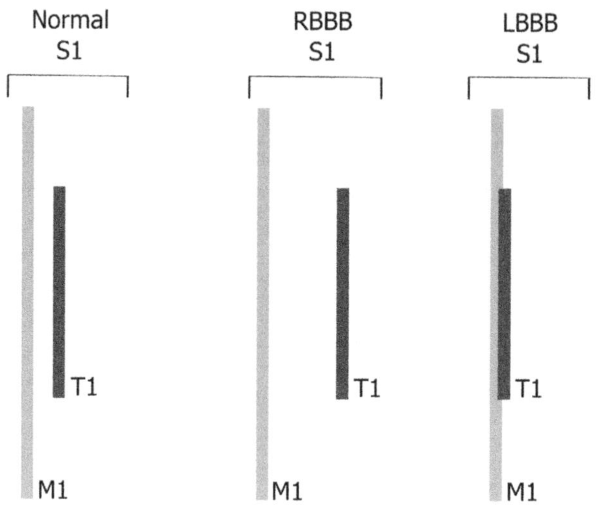

Figure 5.1: Normal and abnormal differences in the components of S1 (M1 and T1).

S2 is caused by closure of the aortic and pulmonic valves at the beginning of isovolumetric ventricular relaxation when ventricular pressure falls below pulmonary and aortic pressure. As aortic pressure (80 mmHg) is far greater than pulmonary artery pressure (10 mmHg), S2 is normally split with two components (A2 and P2) relating to the closure of the aortic and pulmonic valves, respectively. How split A2 and P2 are depend on physiological conditions, primarily the phase of breathing that influences the pulmonary artery pressure. In expiration pulmonary artery pressure is higher, so the pulmonic valve closes earlier and P2 occurs closer to A2. Conversely, during inspiration pulmonary artery pressure falls, so pulmonic valve closing occurs later and A2 and P2 occur further apart (figure 5.2). This physiological splitting can be heard with a stethoscope, but can be further influenced by diseases as listed in table 5.1.

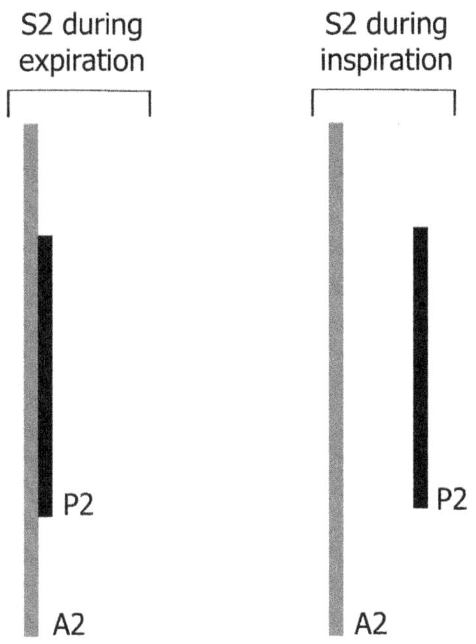

Figure 5.2: Normal splitting of S2 with inspiration.

Changes in S2 splitting and possible underlying causes	
Abnormally wide splitting	- Right ventricle (RV) volume overload (e.g., atrial septal defect) - RV outflow obstruction (e.g., pulmonary stenosis) - RBBB
Narrow splitting	- Pulmonary hypertension - Mild to moderate aortic stenosis
Single S2	- One semilunar valve is absent (e.g., truncus arteriosus, valvular atresia) - Large ventricular septal defect (equal ventricular pressures) - Pulmonary hypertension with equal ventricular pressures
Paradoxical splitting (P2 before A2)	- Severe aortic stenosis - LBBB

Table 5.1: Changes in S2 splitting and possible underlying causes.

S3 is associated with the rapid filling phase of the ventricle (when the AV valves open), about 0.14 to 0.16 seconds after S2 (closure of the aortic and pulmonic valves). The exact cause of the sound is unclear, but a normal S3 occurs as a brief, low-frequency vibration. Previously thought to be an intracardiac sound arising from vibrations in the valve cusps or ventricular wall, more recent studies suggest the sound may be due to the filling ventricular wall hitting the inner chest wall, or it may arise from the ventricular apex as it hits a limitation of its longitudinal expansion.

Common causes of abnormal S3
Dilated cardiomyopathy
Chronic mitral valve regurgitation
Diastolic heart failure
Pregnancy (not pathological sign)
Athletes (not pathological sign)

Table 5.2: Common causes of abnormal S3.

As S3 is a filling sound, an abnormal S3 (higher pitch and referred to as a ventricular gallop) is an important clue to heart failure or volume overload (see table 5.2). The absence of an abnormal S3 does not rule out heart failure, but its presence is a sensitive indicator of ventricular dysfunction. Constriction around the heart (e.g., constrictive pericarditis) may cause an early S3, or "pericardial knock."

S4 is abnormal and is associated with poor ventricular compliance (e.g., ventricular hypertrophy). It occurs during atrial contraction and is associated with the atrial pressure pulse. The sound is thought to be caused by reverberation of the stiffened ventricular wall as blood is propelled into the ventricle from the atrium (hence it is also known as an atrial gallop). S4 and raised end-diastolic ventricular pressure (EDVP) commonly occur together as both are caused by poor ventricular compliance, so S4 tends to be associated with conditions that cause pressure overload (see table 5.3).

Common causes of abnormal S4
Hypertensive heart disease
Aortic stenosis
Hypertrophic cardiomyopathy
Acute phase of myocardial infarction
Acute and severe mitral or aortic regurgitation

Table 5.3: Common causes of abnormal S4.

Ejection Sounds (Clicks)

As S1 and S2 occur during closure of heart valves, pathological conditions can lead to the valves producing a high-frequency "clicking" sound when they open during chamber ejection—hence they can be referred to as ejection sounds and they are pathological.

Aortic ejection sounds usually occur 0.12–0.14 seconds after the Q-wave of the ECG (i.e., after ventricular pressure has risen to exceed aortic pressure). Because of its timing, the "click" produced can be misinterpreted as a split S1. The abnormal opening of the aortic valve is usually caused by a deformed but mobile valve leaflet or aortic root dilation that may be caused by the conditions listed in table 5.4.

Pulmonary ejection sounds occur a little earlier (0.09–0.11 seconds) after the Q-wave as the pulmonary valve opens a little earlier (figure 5.1). It can also be distinguished by the fact that its intensity is diminished during inspiration as increased venous return during inspiration augments the effect of atrial contraction and causes a "gentler" opening of the valve. As with the aortic ejection sounds, pulmonary ejection sounds are associated with deformed valves or pulmonary arterial dilation.

A click occurring in diastole is associated with abnormal opening of either the mitral or tricuspid valve. Similar to systolic clicks, a diastolic click can be misinterpreted as a split S2. The most common cause of diastolic clicks is valvular stenosis of an AV valve.

Aortic	**Pulmonary**
- Aortic stenosis - Bicuspid aortic valve - Aortic regurgitation - Aneurysm in ascending aorta	- Pulmonary stenosis - Pulmonary arterial dilation - Pulmonary hypertension

Table 5.4: Common causes of ejection "clicks."

Heart Murmurs

A murmur is the sound of turbulence associated with abnormal blood flow through a valve or chamber. The turbulent flow produces low-frequency audible sounds that are distinct from heart sounds associated with valve closures. Murmurs can be divided into those caused by valvular defects and those caused by abnormal interchamber flow. Depending on the defect involved, the murmur may occur during diastole and systole, hence distinguishing whether a murmur is diastolic or systolic is a useful first diagnostic step.

Classification of a murmur includes the intensity (Grades 1-6, faintest to loudest), the pitch (high or low), configuration, location, and timing. The timing refers to the onset and duration of the murmur, and the classifications are shown in table 5.5 with some common causes listed there and below.

- **Aortic stenosis** produces a midsystolic murmur that has a crescendo-decrescendo pattern (intensity builds up, then fades). This pattern relates to the level of turbulent flow through the narrowed valve—slow at first as the resistance is overcome, then fading away as blood flow decreases.
- **Mitral/tricuspid regurgitation** produces a holosystolic murmur as the incompetent valve allows a constant turbulent (and reverse) flow from the ventricle back to the atria.
- **Mitral valve prolapse** produces a late-systolic murmur often proceeded by a midsystolic click. The click is caused by tensioning of the chordae tendineae as ventricular pressure increases and the murmur builds up as regurgitation is established.
- **Ventricular septal defect** produces a holosystolic murmur when severe. Turbulent flow through the defect is constant as the left ventricular pressure is higher than right ventricular pressure throughout systole—hence a continuous left-right shunt is established.
- **Aortic regurgitation** produces a "blowing" diastolic murmur that is usually decrescendo. This early diastolic murmur is short because rapidly rising ventricular pressure (due to atrial and aortic contributions) ends the reverse flow from the aorta. In cases when the aortic pressure is high, the regurgitation may be sustained and the murmur becomes pandiastolic.
- **Mitral stenosis** produces a diastolic murmur that starts late as the stenosed valve prevents atria-to-ventricular flow until high atrial pressures are established. The murmur may be preceded by a middiastolic click as the atrial pressure finally "flings" the valve open.

Classification	Description		Possible cause
Early-systolic	Obscures S1 and extends for a variable length in systole but does not extend up to S2		Small ventricular septal defect
Midsystolic	Begins after S1 and ends before A2 or P2. Both S1 and S2 are audible		Aortic stenosis
Holosystolic (a.k.a. pansystolic)	Starts with S1 and extends up to A2 or P2, obscuring both S1 and S2		Ventricular septal defect or AV valve regurgitation
Late-systolic	Starts after S1 and obscures A2 or P2		Mitral valve prolapse
Early-diastolic	Starts with A2 or P2 and extends into diastole for a variable duration		Aortic regurgitation
Middiastolic	Starts after S2 and terminates before S1		Atrial septal defect
Late-diastolic	Starts well after S2 and extends up to the mitral component or to the tricuspid component of S1	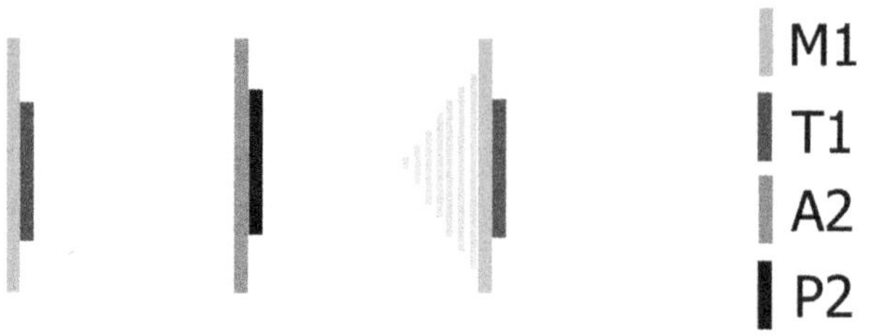	Mitral stenosis

Table 5.5: Classifications of heart murmurs.

References, resources, and further reading

Text

Dornbush, Sean, and Andre E. Turnquest. *Physiology, Heart Sounds*. Treasure Island, FL: StatPearls Publishing, 2022. https://www.ncbi.nlm.nih.gov/books/NBK541010, CC BY 4.0.

Kulkarni, Vivek T., and Leonard S. Lilly. "The Cardiac Cycle: Mechanisms of Heart Sounds and Murmurs." In *Pathophysiology of Heart Disease: A Collaborative Project of Medical Students and Faculty*, 5e edited by Leonard S. Lilly, Chapter 2. Philadelphia: Lippincott Williams & Wilkins, a Wolters Kluwer Business, 2010.

Thomas, Seth L., Joseph Heaton, and Amgad N. Makaryus. *Physiology, Cardiovascular Murmurs*. Treasure Island, FL: StatPearls Publishing, 2022. https://www.ncbi.nlm.nih.gov/books/NBK525958, CC BY 4.0.

Figures

Figure 5.1: Normal and abnormal differences in the components of S1 (M1 and T1). Grey, Kindred. 2022. CC BY 4.0. https://archive.org/details/5.1_20220113

Figure 5.2: Normal splitting of S2 with inspiration. Grey, Kindred. 2022. CC BY 4.0. https://archive.org/details/5.2_20220113

Table 5.5: Classifications of heart murmurs. Grey, Kindred. 2022. CC BY 4.0. https://archive.org/details/5.5_20220113

6. Congenital Heart Disease

Learning Objectives

- Describe the malformations of heart and/or major vascular structures in common congenital heart diseases.
- Determine the flow of blood through the heart, and systemic and pulmonary circulations in common congenital heart diseases.

In this chapter we will look at congenital heart diseases on a disease-by-disease basis. It might also be useful to review your heart embryology as it is highly relevant to the defects we will be looking at.

Atrial Septal Defect (ASD)

Embryology

The most common atrial septal defects arise from:

- Failure of the osteum secundum (most common),
- Excessive resorption of the septum primum, or
- Failure of septum primum to fuse with endocardial cushions (less common).

A patent foramen ovale (20 percent of the population) is not a true ASD as no tissue is missing and the remaining tissue acts as a one-way valve, so a PFO does not have the same pathophysiology as a true ASD. ASDs are common in infants with Down syndrome, as are VSDs.

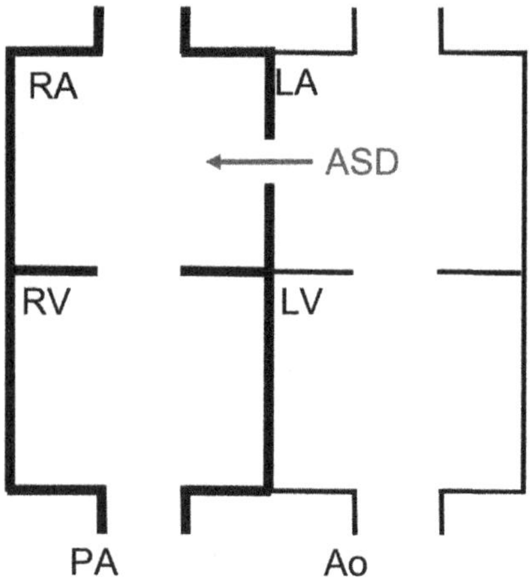

Figure 6.1: Schematic of ASD showing left-right shunt. Thicker lines indicate the presence of volume overload.

Pathophysiology

ASDs allow blood flow between the atria. As the pressure in the left atria is higher than that in the left, blood flows from left to right (figure 6.1). This causes volume overload of the right side of the heart. This excessive load may lead to right ventricular compliance being reduced as remodeling takes place. The reduced compliance can elevate right-side pressure and thereby reduce the left-right shunt.

Ventricular Septal Defect (VSD)

Embryology

Most ventricular septal defects arise from membraneous portion of the septum (70 percent), while others form in the muscular portion (20 percent); less frequently they occur near the aortic or AV valves.

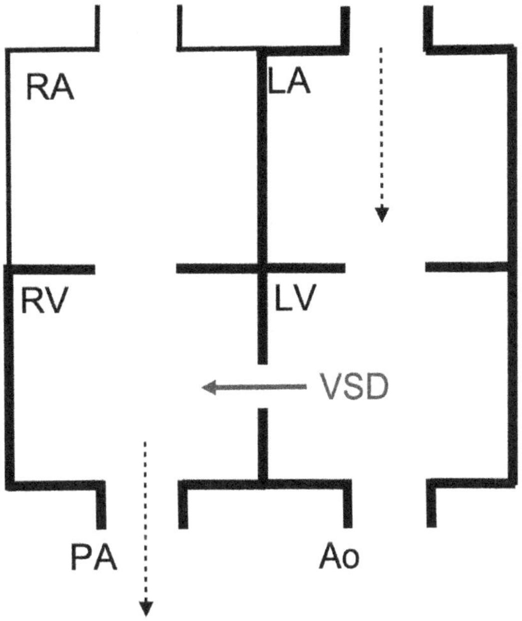

Figure 6.2: Schematic of VSD showing left-right shunt that can lead to volume overload in the RV, LA, LV, and pulmonary circulation. Dotted lines show the recirculation of blood back through the pulmonary circulation. Thicker lines denote volume overload.

Pathophysiology

The manifestations of a VSD depend on the VSD size and the relative resistance of the pulmonary and systemic circulations—all of which will determine the direction of blood flow. During fetal development, the pulmonary and systemic circulations have equivalent resistances, so there may be very little shunting through the VSD, particularly if it is small. After birth, however, the resistance of the pulmonary system falls dramatically, so right ventricular pressure is lower and below left ventricular pressure (which still has to contend with systemic resistance)—consequently a left-right shunt is established. If this shunt is large (depending on the size of the defect), then blood returning from the pulmonary circulation to the left atrium can pass into the left ventricle, through the VSD into the right ventricle and head back into pulmonary circulation to start this loop again (figure 6.2).

When a large VSD is present, the recirculated blood causes volume overload of the right ventricle and the pulmonary circulation and subsequently both chambers of the left heart (figure 6.2). This can eventually cause chamber dilation and lead to heart failure. The extra volume load in the pulmonary circulation can also lead to early onset of pulmonary vascular disease.

Coarctation of the Aorta

Embryology

Coarctation of the aorta (figure 6.3) is a constriction of the aortic lumen, usually close to the ductus. The cause is unclear, but low flow through the left heart and aorta flow during development may cause the defect (no flow, no grow).

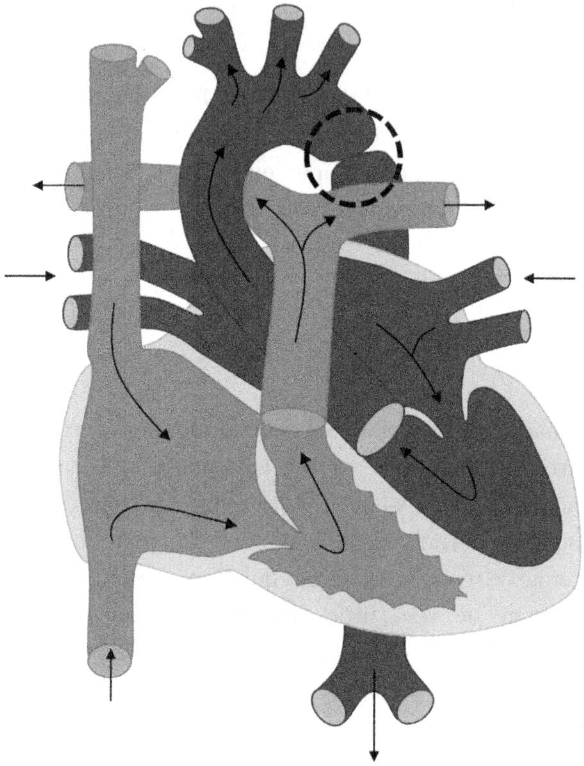

Figure 6.3: Coarctation of the aorta (circled).

Pathophysiology

The diminished lumen causes increased afterload on the left ventricle. Vessels branching off the aorta before the coarctation can receive normal blood flow, so the head (carotid) and upper extremities (subclavian) are usually properly perfused whereas branching arteries after the coarctation may be underperfused. Consequently, differential cyanosis is a possible manifestation.

Tetralogy of Fallot (ToF)

Embryology

In Tetralogy of Fallot (ToF) the outflow tract (infundibular) portion of the interventricular septum is displaced. This single defect leads to four defects:

1. Subvalvular pulmonic stenosis, because of the displaced infundibular septum (#1, figure 6.4),
2. Right ventricular hypertrophy caused by the pulmonic stenosis (#2, figure 6.4),
3. VSD—caused by malalignment of the interventricular septum (#3, figure 6.4), and
4. Overriding aorta that receives blood from both ventricles (#4, figure 6.4).

Other defects can be associated with ToF, but the defects listed above lead this to be the most common form of cyanotic congenital heart disease.

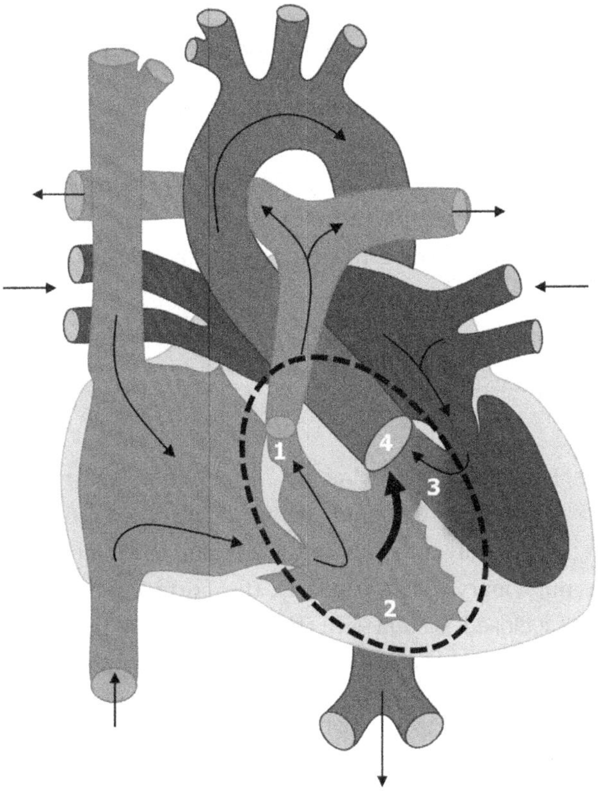

Figure 6.4: Tetralogy of Fallot with 1) pulmonic stenosis, 2) RV hypertrophy, 3) VSD, and 4) overriding aorta.

Pathophysiology

The high resistance of the stenosed pulmonic valve (#1, figure 6.4) causes the blood in the right ventricle to exit through VSD (#3, figure 6.4) and enter the left ventricle forming a right-left shunt, bypassing the pulmonary circulation. Consequently blood with venous PO_2 enters the systemic circulation and hypoxemia/cyanosis results. The degree of hypoxemia/cyanosis that occurs depends on the degree of pulmonic stenosis.

Transposition of the Great Arteries

Embryology

Although not completely understood, it is thought that failure of the aortic-pulmonary septum to spiral during development results in the great vessels coming off the wrong ventricles—the aorta exits the right, and the pulmonary artery exits the left. Other theories exist.

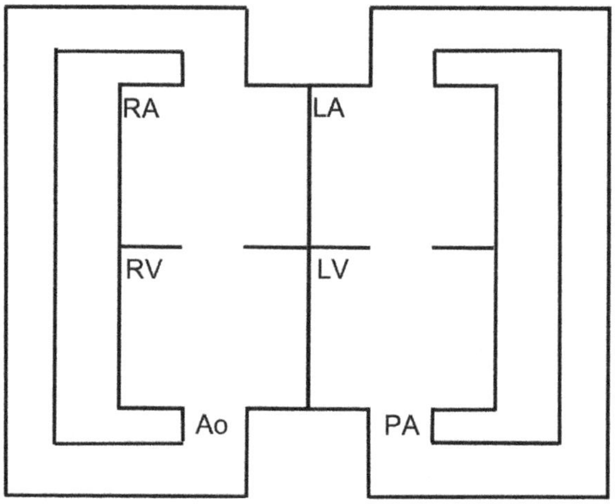

Figure 6.5: Schematic of transposition of the great vessels (aorta off of the right, pulmonary artery off of the left) forming two separate, looped circulations.

Pathophysiology

The placement of the pulmonary artery on the left means left ventricular blood is pumped up to pulmonary circulation, only to return to the left side of the heart via the pulmonary veins. Similarly, the aorta on the right forms a closed-system with the right ventricle pumping into the systemic circulation, only for it to return to the right atrium via the vena cava (see figure 6.5). So how is this compatible with life? In short, it is not. Embryonic development can continue because the two looped circulations can mix at the ductus arteriosus and foramen ovale of the fetal circulation. But after birth these shunts between the two circulations MUST be artificially maintained, or the patient must be "fortunate" enough to also have a VSD for mixing to take place.

Patent Ductus Arteriosus

Embryology

The ductus arteriosus is part of the fetal circulation allowing blood in the pulmonary artery to bypass the nonfunctional, high resistance lungs and instead traverse into the aorta and systemic circulation. The ductus should close at birth, and failure to do so leaves a patent ductus arteriosus (PDA).

Pathophysiology

In utero, the high resistance of the pulmonary circulation ensures that blood is diverted through the ductus arteriosis into the aorta. However, at birth there is a dramatic fall in the resistance of the pulmonary circulation as the lungs inflate. The pressure gradient across the ductus is consequently reversed (low on the pulmonary side, high on the systemic), so if the ductus remains open blood will flow from the aorta to the pulmonary artery (i.e., the opposite direction to fetal circulation) (figure 6.6).

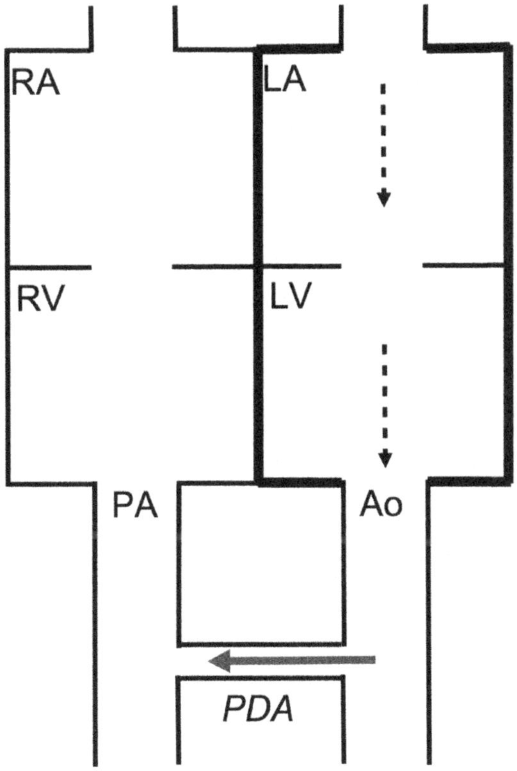

Figure 6.6: Schematic of PDA with flow from the aorta to the pulmonary artery. Thicker lines denote volume overload.

The consequences of this are that a greater volume of blood reenters the pulmonary circulation, the left atria, and the left ventricle. Consequently the compartments of the left heart can eventually fail through volume overload. When the left heart fails, the shunt through the PDA can be reversed, and desaturated blood destined for the pulmonary circulation can end up passing through the PDA to the aorta instead—this reversal later in life is called Eisenmenger syndrome. In Eisenmenger's the upper extremities receive uncontaminated, saturated blood, as their branching arteries are upstream of the desaturated blood entering the aorta at the PDA. Not so for the lower extremities whose arteries branch after the PDA and so receive low oxygen blood. Hence in Eisenmenger syndrome patients, only the feet are cyanosed.

Atrioventricular Canal

Embryology

Complete AV canal defect is a result of complete failure of fusion between endocardial cushions. It is characterized by a primum atrial septal defect (#1, figure 6.7) that is contiguous with a ventricular septal defect (#4 in figure 6.7) and a malformed or common AV valve. Although several forms of this defect exist, this complete form is effectively a single chambered heart.

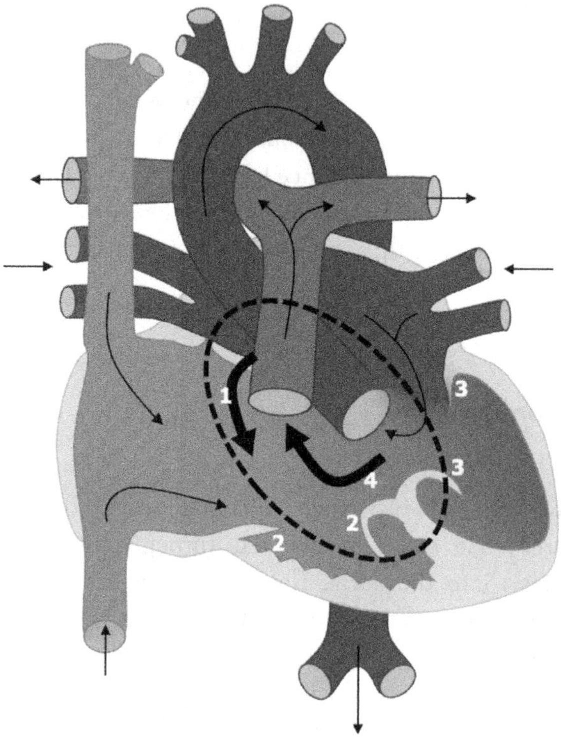

Figure 6.7: AV Canal with 1) ASD, 2&3) AV *valve defects, and* 4) VSD.

Pathophysiology

The malformed valves allow regurgitation, and the unrestricted interventricular communication allow a profound left-right shunt. This leads to volume overload in the pulmonary circulation, and heart failure will be produced if there is no correction. Pulmonary artery hypertension (PAH) and premature development of pulmonary vascular obstructive disease are other common outcomes.

Truncus Arteriosus

Embryology

Failed development of the truncoconal septum that normally leads to separation of the pulmonary artery and aorta leads to truncus arteriosus (TA). This condition leads to a single vessel with a single (often incompetent) valve positioned above the ventricular septum (see figure 6.8).

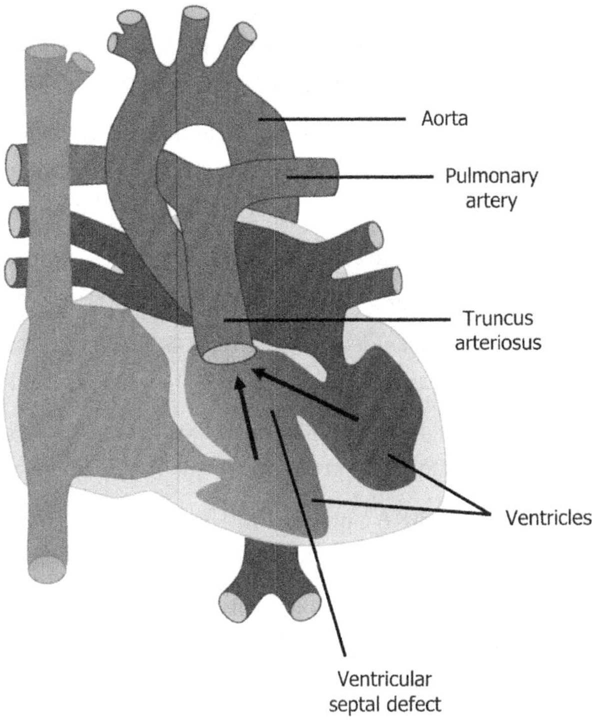

Figure 6.8: Truncus arteriosus.

Pathophysiology

The underlying issues with TA are 1) mixing of blood from the left (saturated) and right heart (unsaturated), and 2) the common valve can allow regurgitation. *In utero* the high pulmonary vascular resistance means most blood exiting the heart goes through the aorta and cardiac output is rarely affected. At birth mild cyanosis can be produced by the mixing of blood from the left and right heart, but as pulmonary vascular resistance remains high in the first few days of life, cardiac output my be maintained. As pulmonary vascular resistance continues to fall in the first few weeks of life, a significant left-right shunt can become established as more left ventricular blood finds it "easier" to ascend up the pulmonary artery. Similar to a VSD, this leads to volume overload in the pulmonary circulation and eventually heart failure. The heart failure has a more rapid onset in TA than VSD if the common valve allows regurgitation. The regurgitation lowers end-diastolic ventricular volumes, so cardiac work to maintain cardiac output increases and promotes myocardial ischemia. Add to this the left-right shunt (as seen in VSD) and heart failure is more likely.

References, resources, and further reading

Text

Bhansali, Suneet, and Colin Phoon. *Truncus Arteriosis*. Treasure Island, FL: StatPearls Publishing, 2022. https://www.ncbi.nlm.nih.gov/books/NBK534774/, CC BY 4.0.

Cunningham, Jonathan W., and David W. Brown. "Congenital Heart Disease." In *Pathophysiology of Heart Disease: A Collaborative Project of Medical Students and Faculty*, edited by Leonard S. Lilly, Chapter 16. Philadelphia: Lippincott Williams & Wilkins, a Wolters Kluwer Business, 2012.

Dakkak, Wael, and Tony I. Oliver. *Ventricular Septal Defect*. Treasure Island, FL: StatPearls Publishing, 2022. https://www.ncbi.nlm.nih.gov/books/NBK470330/, CC BY 4.0.

Diaz-Frias, Josua, and Melissa Guillaume. *Tetralogy of Fallot*. Treasure Island, FL: StatPearls Publishing, 2022. https://www.ncbi.nlm.nih.gov/books/NBK513288/, CC BY 4.0.

Gillam-Krakauer, Maria, and Kunal Mahajan. *Patent Ductus Ateriosus*. Treasure Island, FL: StatPearls Publishing, 2022. https://www.ncbi.nlm.nih.gov/books/NBK430758/, CC BY 4.0.

Law, Mark A., and Vijai S. Tivakaran. *Coarctation of the Aorta*. Treasure Island, FL: StatPearls Publishing, 2022. https://www.ncbi.nlm.nih.gov/books/NBK430913/, CC BY 4.0.

Menillo, Alexandra M., Lawrence S. Lee, and Anthony L. Pearson-Shaver. *Atrial Septal Defect*. Treasure Island, FL: StatPearls Publishing, 2022. https://www.ncbi.nlm.nih.gov/books/NBK535440/, CC BY 4.0.

Szymanski, Michael W., Sheila M. Moore, Stacy M. Kritzmire, and Amandeep Goyal. *Transposition of the Great Arteries*. Treasure Island, FL: StatPearls Publishing, 2022. https://www.ncbi.nlm.nih.gov/books/NBK430758/, CC BY 4.0.

Umapathi, Krishna Kishore, and Pradyumna Agasthi. *Atrioventricular Canal Defects*. Treasure Island, FL: StatPearls Publishing, 2022. https://www.ncbi.nlm.nih.gov/books/NBK557511/, CC BY 4.0.

Figures

Figure 6.1: Schematic of ASD showing left-right shunt. Thicker lines indicate presence of volume overload. Binks, Andrew. 2022. CC BY 4.0.

Figure 6.2: Schematic of VSD showing left-right shunt that can lead to volume overload in the RV, LA, LV and pulmonary circulation. Binks, Andrew. 2022. CC BY 4.0.

Figure 6.3: Coarctation of the aorta (circled). Grey, Kindred. 2022. CC BY 4.0. https://archive.org/details/6.3_20220113

Figure 6.4: Tetraology of fallot with (1) pulmonic stenosis, (2) RV hypertrophy, (3) VSD, and (4) overriding aorta. Grey, Kindred. 2022. CC BY 4.0. https://archive.org/details/6.4_20220113

Figure 6.5: Schematic of transposition of the great vessels (aorta off the right, pulmonary artery off the left) forming two separate, looped circulations. Binks, Andrew. 2022. CC BY 4.0.

Figure 6.6: Schematic of PDA with flow from aorta to pulmonary artery. Binks, Andrew. 2022. CC BY 4.0.

Figure 6.7: AV Canal with (1) ASD, (2&3) AV valve defects, and (4) VSD. Grey, Kindred. 2022. CC BY 4.0. https://archive.org/details/6.7_20220113

Figure 6.8: Truncus arteriosus. Grey, Kindred. 2022. CC BY 4.0. https://archive.org/details/6.8-copy

7. Ischemic Heart Disease

Learning Objectives

- Distinguish between different degrees of myocardial ischemia and their pathophysiological impact.
- Determine the location of infarcted myocardium using a 12-lead ECG.

Atherosclerosis is the pathological process by which the structure of an artery is disrupted through the deposition of cholesterol with the intima of the wall. Initially starting as a "fatty streak" the accumulating cholesterol can lead to the formation of an atherosclerotic plaque with a more complex, but ultimately less stable, structure. During this process the endothelium becomes dysfunctional and the growing plaque can impinge on the lumen of the vessel causing reduced blood flow to the downstream tissue and cause ischemia. When the atherosclerotic plaque forms within the coronary arteries (coronary artery disease, or CAD), the subsequent myocardial ischemia can lead to acute coronary syndromes and ST segment elevation MI, or STEMI. When present in other circulations, atherosclerosis can contribute to stroke, peripheral arterial disease, aortic aneurysms, renal artery disease, and mesenteric ischemia.

The process by which atherosclerotic plaques form is summarized in figure 7.1, but there are four fundamental stages:

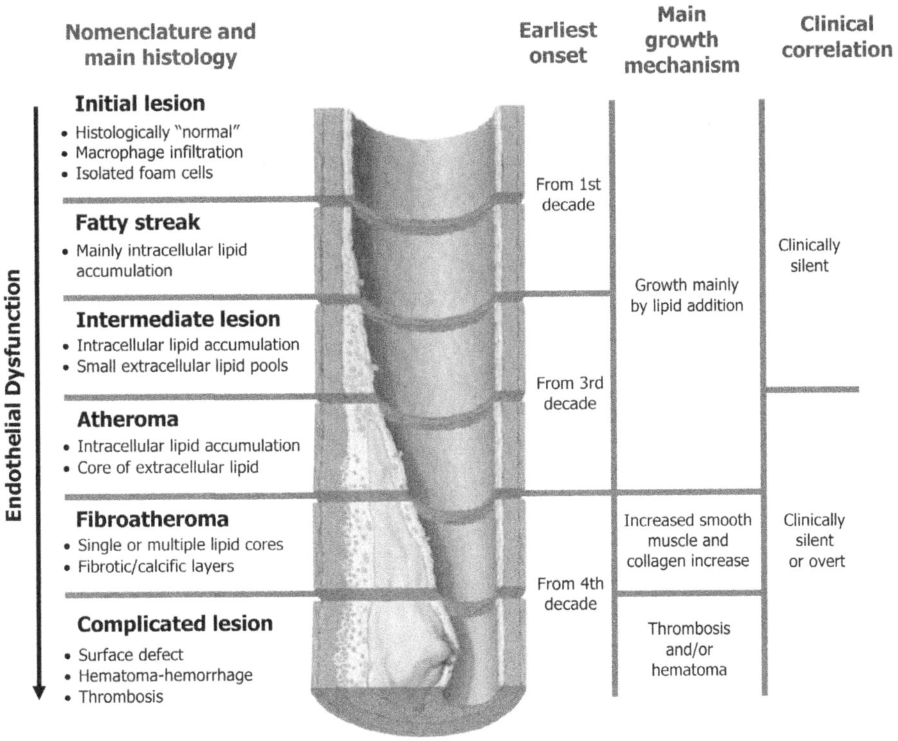

Figure 7.1: Sequences in progression of atherosclerosis.

1. **Endothelial cell injury.** The process is likely initiated by endothelial damage. The potential causes of this damage are numerous and involve any toxin to which the endothelium is exposed. This is reflected in the risk factors for CAD such as tobacco use, diabetes, and dyslipidemia, all of which can cause endothelial damage. As well as chemical insults to the endothelium, excessive physical force can also cause damage and likely contributes to the correlation of CAD and hypertension.
2. **Lipoprotein deposition.** The damaged endothelium allows entry of cholesterol (LDL) into the vessel wall, whereupon it is oxidized (mLDL) and results in an inflammatory response that includes expression of MCP-1 (monocyte chemattractant protein-1) that attracts monocytes from the bloodstream. The monocytes enter the wall, and the mLDL promotes their transition to macrophage. The macrophages ingest the mLDL to become "foam cells" that form the fatty streak.
3. **Inflammatory reaction.** As well as consuming the mLDL, the macrophages release cytokines that attract other white blood cells (including T-lymphcytes) to the vessel wall through endothelial expression of adhesion molecules (e.g., ICAM-1, VCAM-1, E-selectin, and P-selectin).
4. **Smooth muscle cell cap formation and weakening.** The T-lymphocytes release cytokines that promote migration of smooth muscle cells to the surface of the plaque that create a "fibrous cap." This cap is initially thick and therefore stable. However, continued arrival and action of T-lymphocytes subsequently weaken the plaque's structural integrity as they penetrate the cap and release IFN-γ that inhibits collagen production, while activated macrophages simultaneously destroy the cap's collagen. Calcification of the plaque also reduces its integrity. The weakened plaque is now more prone to rupture and inducing formation of a thrombus (see figure 7.2).

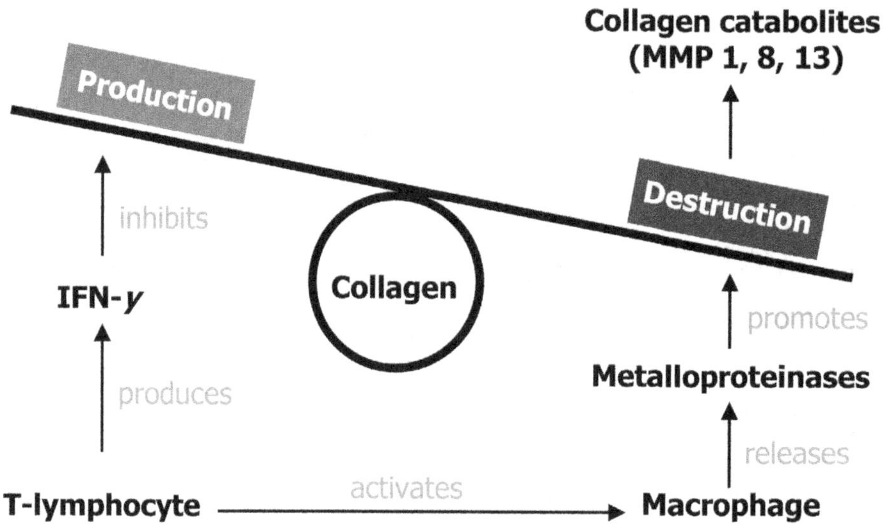

Figure 7.2: Weakening of an atherosclerotic plaque by T-lymphocytes.

Types of Myocardial Ischemia and Infarction

The degree of occlusion caused by the plaque and the oxygen demand of the myocardium determine the degree of ischemia that can develop. Arterial occlusion tends not to be a significant factor until the lumen is occluded by about 70 percent. Vascular occlusion may also be masked by formation of anastomoses (new vessels that bypass the occlusion). Rupture of the plaque and formation of a thrombus can drastically and quickly reduce the lumen and blood flow. The degree and duration of ischemia determine the type of acute coronary syndrome that occurs and the clinical impact. Mild or brief ischemia can lead to angina pectoris with no permanent tissue damage, but when ischemia is prolonged then myocardial infarction becomes more likely, and significant changes in ECG and release of cardiac enzymes are seen.

Stable and unstable angina pectoris

While not considered an acute coronary syndrome, stable angina is pain associated with periods of myocardial ischemia, usually associated with exertion and an increase in myocardial oxygen demand that is unmeet because of insufficient tissue perfusion. The inadequate perfusion is most commonly caused by coronary artery disease (vessel occlusion). Stable angina is predictable and regular, and resolves when the myocardial oxygen demand is reduced (i.e., cessation of exercise).

Unstable angina is more serious and may be an unpredictable exacerbation of anginal pain that had previously been stable. It may occur at rest or lower than usual levels of exertion. Unstable angina is part of the acute coronary syndrome spectrum and may reflect rupture of a plaque that has led to thrombosis. The ECG in unstable angina may show hyperacute T-waves, flattening of the T-waves, inverted T-waves, and ST depression. Without the presence of myocardial damage, unstable angina is not associated with elevated cardiac enzymes (e.g., troponin). Continued or worsening stenosis of the coronary artery leads to tissue infarction and more clinically significant elements of acute coronary syndrome.

Non-ST segment elevation myocardial infarction

With non-ST segment elevation myocardial infarction (NSTEMI), there is necrosis of the myocardium. Although, as the name suggests, there is no consistent ST segment elevation in a NSTEMI, other ECG changes may be seen. These include transient ST elevation, ST depression, or new T-wave inversions. The lysing myocytes release their contents including enzymes that can be used as biomarkers of the necrotic event. Presence of elevated cardiac enzymes distinguishes NSTEMI from unstable angina, but denotes myocardial damage and a poorer prognosis. There are several cardiac enzymes that can be detected (myoglobin, creatine kinase, and troponin I), and each has a different timeline from onset of infarction (figure 7.3). But because of improvements in test sensitivity, the test enzyme of choice is troponin I.

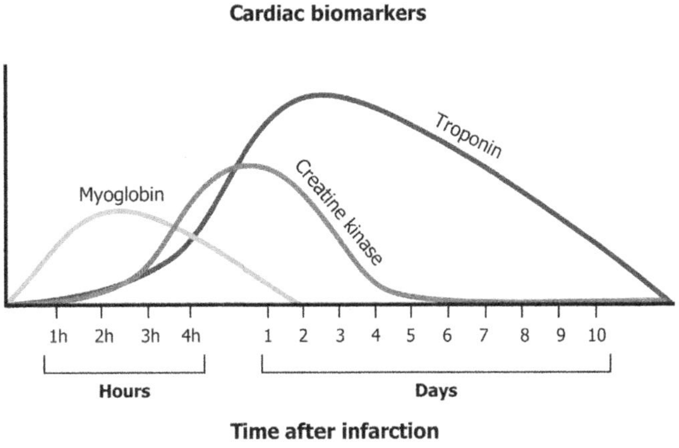

Figure 7.3: Timeline of cardiac biomarkers after a myocardial infarction.

Troponin

Troponin I is a normal protein important in the contractile apparatus of the cardiac myocyte. It is released into the circulation about three to four hours after MI and are still detectable for ten days afterward. The long half-life allows for the late diagnosis of MI but makes it difficult to detect reinfarction (a major complication associated with new thrombus formation during stent placement). Although there are a number causes for troponin elevation unrelated to MI, troponin elevation is much more sensitive and specific than myoglobin and even creatine kinase.

ST segment elevation myocardial infarction

ST segment elevation myocardial infarction (STEMI) most often results from complete occlusion of a major epicardial vessel. The resultant myocardial infarction raises cardiac enzymes measured in the blood (as with NSTEMI), but is accompanied by an ST segment elevation on the 12-lead ECG. This is the most serious of the acute coronary syndromes.

Pathophysiology of a STEMI

The most common cause of a STEMI is rupture of an atherosclerotic plaque. The continued degradation and calcification of the fibrous cap results in it breaking and spilling its contents into the bloodstream. Tissue factor within the necrotic core instigates the coagulation cascade when it is exposed to the blood and a thrombus is formed and the vessel is occluded. Plaques rupture most frequently at their "shoulder," the thin peripheral edges where proteolytic and apoptotic activity are highest and mechanical forces are most effective. The tissue downstream from the occlusion experiences ischemia and then infarcts. The impact on cardiac function and output depends on the site and extent of the infarcted tissue. For example, if a significant section of the left ventricular wall is involved, then the fall in cardiac output may be catastrophic, or if the papillary muscles of a valve are included, the valve may become incompetent and allow regurgitation.

Physical Exam of a STEMI

The physical examination findings may include elevated heart rate and blood pressure due to increased sympathetic tone. However, if cardiac function is severely impacted because of the size or location of the infarction, cardiogenic shock may result with a fall in blood pressure. The insufficient ATP production in the ischemic region means the interaction of actin and myosin in the cardiac myocytes cannot be broken and the muscle cannot relax. An S4 heart sound (figure 7.4) occurs when the noncompliant, stiffened left ventricle vibrates when blood enters from the atrium. The S4 sound is also known as an atrial gallop—not because the sound comes from the ventricle, but because it is associated with atrial contraction (and ventricular filling). If the infarction involves an impact of the papillary muscle function, the associated valve will fail and the regurgitation will cause a holosystolic murmur. A STEMI in the left ventricle sufficient to cause congestion and a rise in left-ventricular and end-diastolic pressure can lead to rises in left atrial and pulmonary pressure; this may be heard on the lung exam as rales due to the transient pulmonary edema.

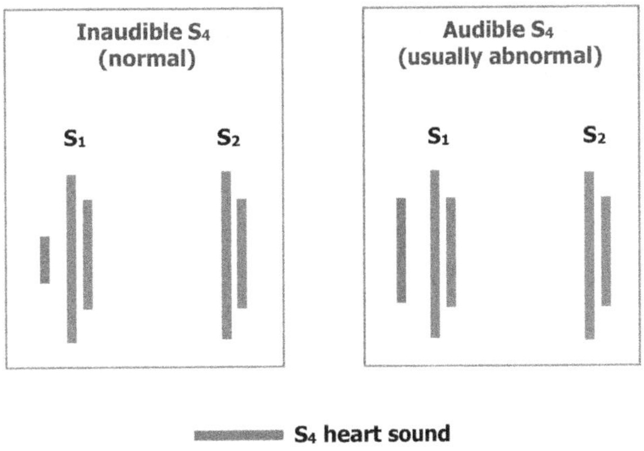

Figure 7.4: Comparison of audible and inaudible S4 sounds.

Diagnosis of a STEMI

As mentioned above the two most important tools for diagnosing a STEMI are the ECG and the presence of cardiac enzymes that have been released into the bloodstream. Figure 7.4 shows the time line of myoglobin, creatine kinase, and troponin elevations after an infarction. Using the values of all three enzymes allowed the history of an infarction to be generated, but amazing improvements in the sensitivity of the troponin I test have allowed it to become the gold standard because of its specificity to the myocardium.

Changes in ECG

The first ECG sign to arise during a STEMI are "hyperacute T-waves" (figure 7.5). These T-waves are taller than normal and caused by the release of intracellular potassium from lysing cells and the consequent hyperkalemia in the surrounding tissue. Hyperacute T-waves are not often seen clinically because they occur so early in the event and prior to the patient's arrival in the hospital. Subsequent ECG stages are more commonly observed, and these include the ST elevation.

Determining which ECG leads show the ST elevation allow for the location of the infarcted tissue to be determined and provide insight into which coronary vessel is effected. How the leads of a twelve-lead ECG relate to the coronary vessels is summarized in figure 7.6. The following looks at the characteristic ECG changes in relation to location in a bit more detail (tip: relate back to figure 7.6 as you read the next sections).

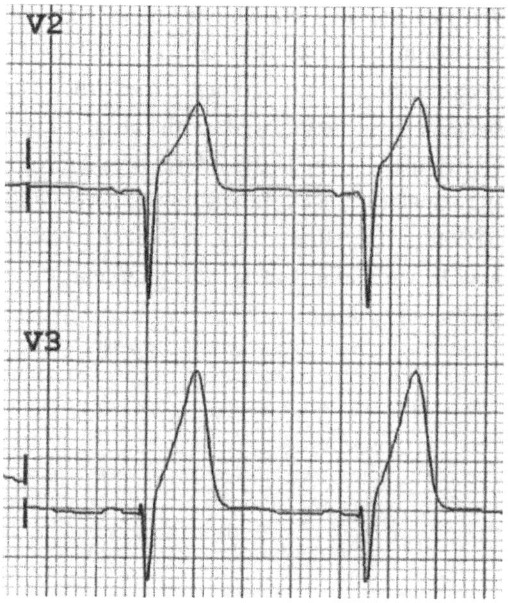

Figure 7.5: Hyperacute T-waves associated with an early myocardial infarction.

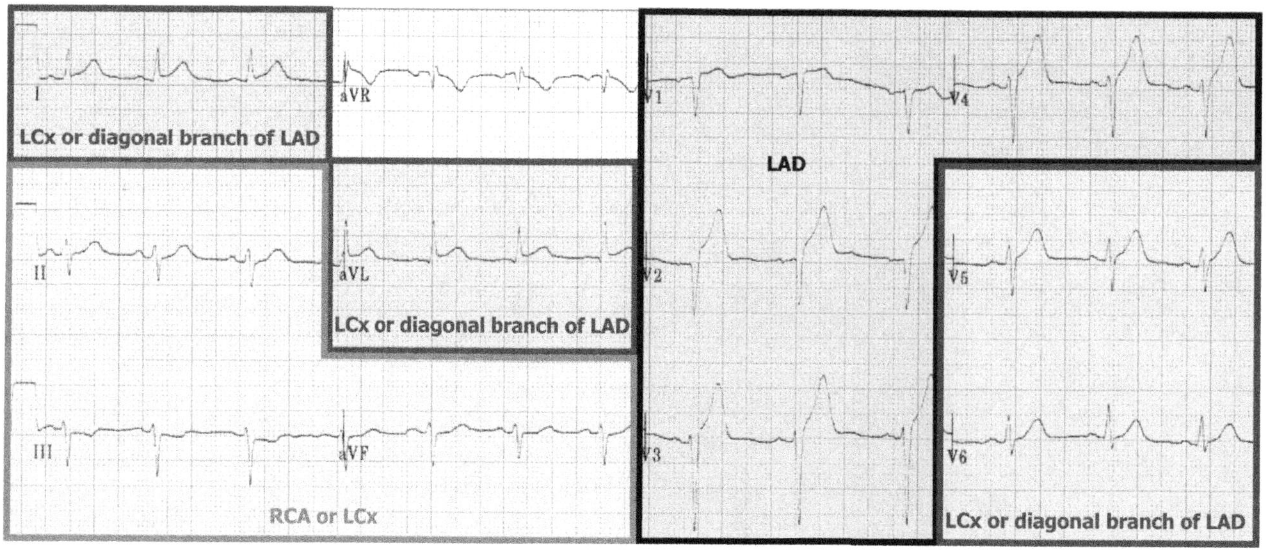

Figure 7.6: Which leads look at which coronary vessels? LCx = left circumflex, LAD = left anterior descending, RCA = right coronary artery.

Anterior wall myocardial infarctions (AWMI)

The anterior wall is affected when the left anterior descending coronary artery becomes occluded. Additional involvement of lateral and septal regions is indicative of the left main coronary artery being involved. Inclusion of these regions is termed an extensive anterior infarction. The ECG shows ST segment elevation in leads V3 and V4 (the anterior leads), seen as a raised J-point (see figure 7.7). A reciprocal ST depression will be seen in leads II, III, and aVF (the inferior leads). If the extent of the infarction is large, the elevated ST segment may been seen in the lateral and septal leads. The elevated ST segment is also associated in a change in shape of the T-wave as it becomes broader and loses its concave shape on the downward section. This broad T-wave can be higher as well as the ST elevation progresses, and its height can surpass the R-wave. These morphological changes result in a T-wave that looks like a tombstone (see figure 7.7).

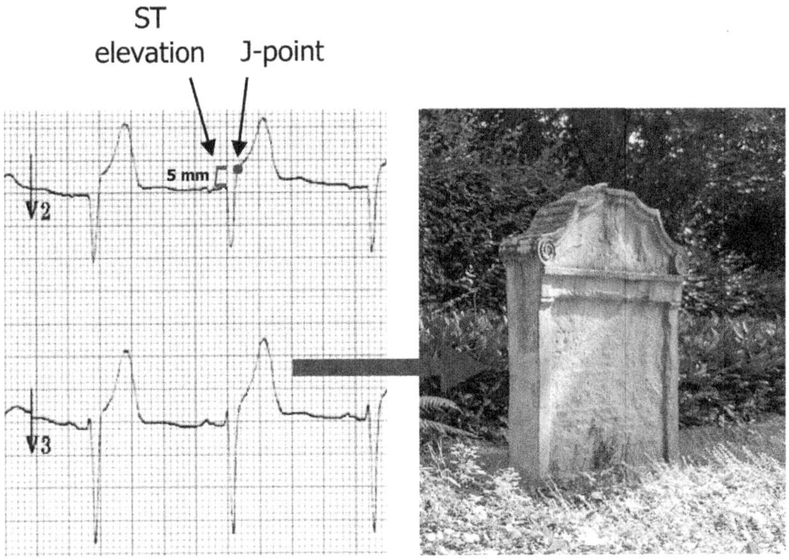

Figure 7.7: An ECG showing an anterior wall infarction with the characteristic "tombstoning" of the T-wave.

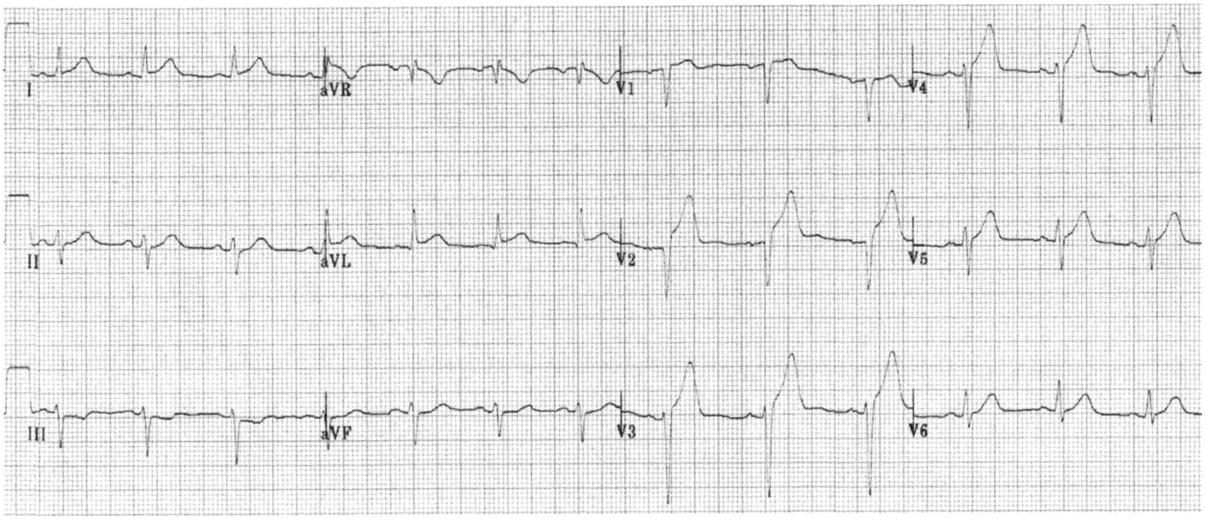

Figure 7.8: AWMI.

Inferior wall myocardial infarction (IWMI)

Occlusion of the right coronary artery is the usual culprit for an inferior wall myocardial infarction (IWMI), which may be severe enough to extend to posterior regions. The ECG findings of an acute inferior myocardial infarction (figure 7.9) will be an ST segment elevation in leads II, III, and aVF (the inferior leads) and reciprocal depression in lead aVL (a lateral lead); without the reciprocal depression in aVL, alternative causes of ST segment elevation in the inferior leads should be considered (e.g., pericarditis). Because the right coronary artery perfuses the SA node, bradycardia may occur. An inferior MI can have multiple potential complications, including cardiogenic shock, atrioventricular block, or ventricular fibrillation, and can be fatal.

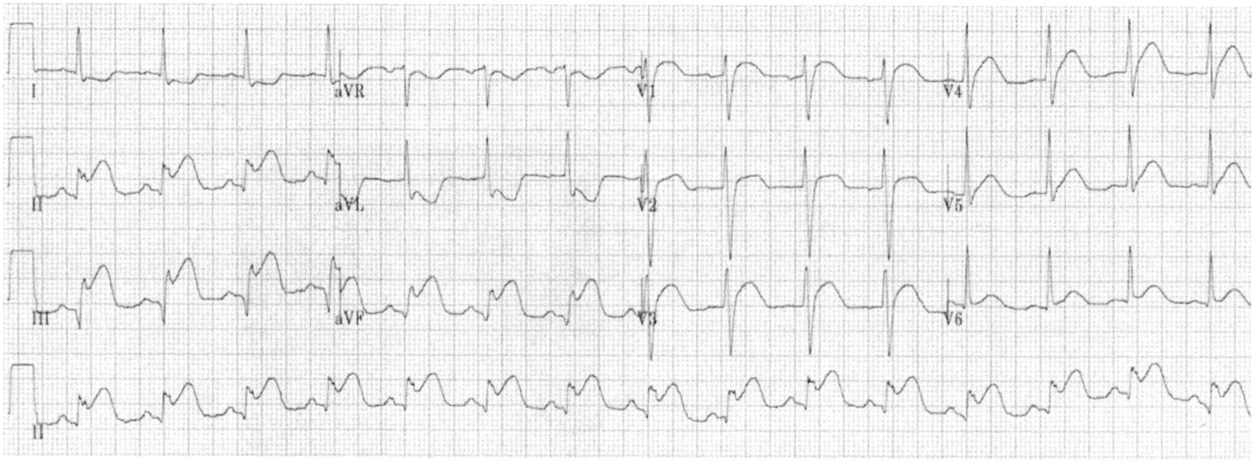

Figure 7.9: IWMI.

Posterior wall myocardial infarction (PWMI)

Most posterior myocardial infarctions occur with occlusion of the posterior descending artery (which in most people is a branch of the right coronary artery); because of the shared supply, a posterior infarction is often accompanied by an IWMI. The ECG findings include ST segment elevation in V7–V9 (the posterior leads that are placed on the posterior axillary line, not shown in figure 7.11) and ST depression in V1–V4 (the septal and anterior leads, shown in figure 7.10). If an IWMI is also present then there will be an ST elevation in leads II, III, and aVF (the inferior leads). A twelve-lead ECG showing a posterior wall infarction is shown in figure 7.11.

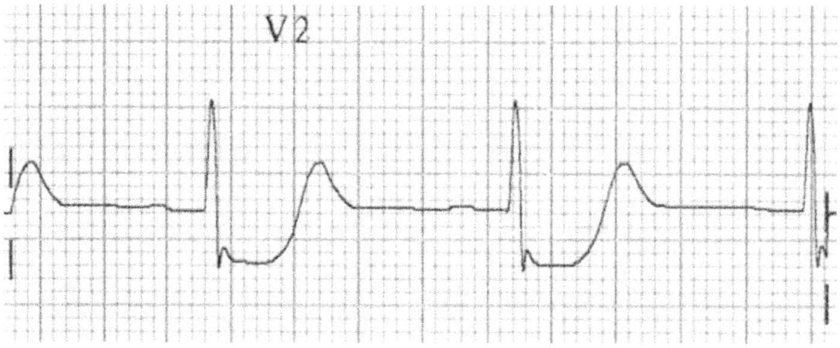

Figure 7.10: Typical appearance of posterior infarction in V2.

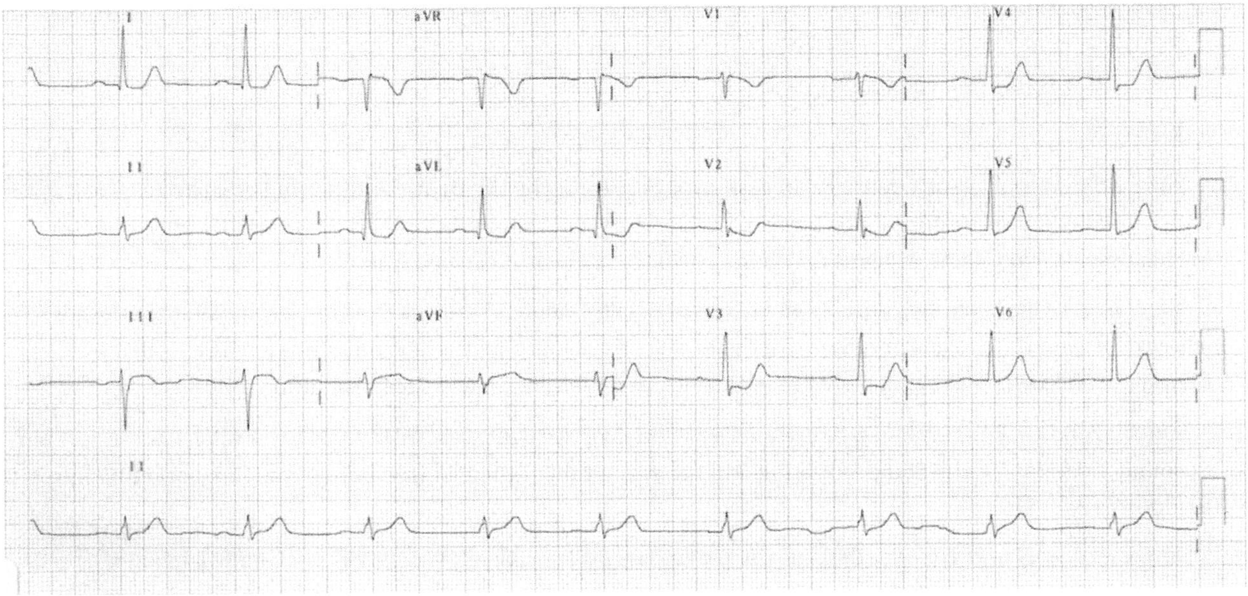

Figure 7.11: Posterior wall MI.

The location of the infarction, leads showing ST elevation and depression, and the involved coronary artery are summarized in table 7.1.

Infarction	**ST Elevation**	**ST Depression**	**Coronary artery**
Anterior wall	V3 and V4	II, III, aVF	Left anterior descending
Inferior wall	II, III, aVF	aVL	Right
Posterior wall	V7-V9	V1-V4	Posterior descending

Table 7.1: Location of the infarction, leads showing ST elevation and depression, and the involved coronary artery.

References, resources, and further reading

Text

Rhee, June-Wha, Sabatine, Marc S., and Leonard S. Lilly. “Ischemic Heart Disease.” In *Pathophysiology of Heart Disease: A Collaborative Project of Medical Students and Faculty*, 5e, edited by Leonard S. Lilly, Chapter 6. Philadelphia: Lippincott Williams & Wilkins, a Wolters Kluwer Business, 2010.

Rhee, June-Wha, Sabatine, Marc S., and Leonard S. Lilly. “Acute Coronary Syndromes.” In *Pathophysiology of Heart Disease: A Collaborative Project of Medical Students and Faculty*, 5e, edited by Leonard S. Lilly, Chapter 7. Philadelphia: Lippincott Williams & Wilkins, a Wolters Kluwer Business, 2010.

Surawicz, Borys, Rory Childers, Barbara J. Deal, and Leonard S. Gettes. “AHA/ACCF/HRS Recommendations for the Standardization and Interpretation of the Electrocardiogram.” *Circulation* 119, no. 10 (2009): e235–e240.

Surawicz, Borys, and Timothy Knilans. *Chou's Electrocardiography in Practice*, 6th ed. Philadelphia: Saunders, 2008.

Figures

Figure 7.1: Sequences in progression of atherosclerosis. Grey, Kindred. 2022. CC BY-SA 4.0. Added Npatchett. “Late Complications of Atherosclerosis.” 2015, from WikimediaCommons, CC BY-SA 4.0. https://archive.org/details/7.1_20220113

Figure 7.2: Weakening of an atherosclerotic plaque by T-lymphocytes. Grey, Kindred. 2022. CC BY 4.0. https://archive.org/details/7.3_20220113

Figure 7.3: Timeline of cardiac biomarkers after a myocardial infarction. Grey, Kindred. 2022. CC BY 4.0. https://archive.org/details/7.3_20220113_202201

Figure 7.4: Comparison of audible and inaudible S4 sounds. Grey, Kindred. 2022. CC BY 4.0. https://archive.org/details/7.2_20220113_202201

Figure 7.5: Hyperacute T-waves associated with an early myocardial infarction. Burns, Ed, and Robert Buttner. Prinzmetal Angina Figure, *T Wave*. Life in the Fast Lane, 2021. https://litfl.com/t-wave-ecg-library/, CC BY-NC-SA 4.0.

Figure 7.6: Which leads look at which coronary vessels? LCx = left circumflex, LAD = left anterior descending, RCA = right coronary. Grey, Kindred. 2022. CC BY-NC-SA 4.0. Added Burns, Ed, and Robert Buttner. Example 1, *Anterior Myocardial Infarction*. Life in the Fast Lane, 2022. https://litfl.com/anterior-myocardial-infarction-ecg-library, CC BY-NC-SA 4.0. https://archive.org/details/7.6_20220113

Figure 7.7: An ECG showing a anterior wall infarction with the characteristic ‘tombstoning’ of the T-wave. Grey, Kindred. 2022. CC BY-NC-SA 4.0. Added Burns, Ed, and Robert Buttner. Example 1, *Anterior Myocardial Infarction*. Life in the Fast Lane, 2022. https://litfl.com/anterior-myocardial-infarction-ecg-library, CC BY-NC-SA 4.0. Added Rabich, Dietmar. “Lüdinghausen, Jüdischer Friedhof — 2013 — 2855.” 2013, from WikimediaCommons, CC BY-NC-SA 4.0. https://archive.org/details/7.6_20220113_202201

Figure 7.8: AWMI. Burns, Ed, and Robert Buttner. Example 1, *Anterior Myocardial Infarction*. Life in the Fast Lane, 2022. https://litfl.com/anterior-myocardial-infarction-ecg-library, CC BY-NC-SA 4.0.

Figure 7.9: IWMI. Buttner, Robert, and Ed Burns. Example 3, *Inferior STEMI*. Life in the Fast Lane, 2021. https://litfl.com/inferior-stemi-ecg-library, CC BY-NC-SA 4.0.

Figure 7.10: Typical appearance of posterior infarction in V2. Burns, Ed. Typical Appearance of Posterior Infarction in V2 Figure, *Posterior Myocardial Infarction*. Life in the Fast Lane, 2021. https://litfl.com/posterior-myocardial-infarction-ecg-library, CC BY-NC-SA 4.0.

Figure 7.11: Posteror wall MI. Burns, Ed. Example 2a, *Posterior Myocardial Infarction*. Life in the Fast Lane, 2021. https://litfl.com/posterior-myocardial-infarction-ecg-library, CC BY-NC-SA 4.0.

Made in the USA
Coppell, TX
04 November 2026

11287989R00044